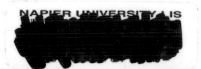

Advanced Nursing Series
MODELS, THEORIES AND CONCEPTS

In Preparation:
RESEARCH AND ITS APPLICATION

Advanced Nursing Series

MODELS, THEORIES AND CONCEPTS

Edited by

JAMES P. SMITH

OBE, BSC (Soc), MSc, DER, SRN, RNT
BTA Certificate, FRCN, FRSH

Editor of the *Journal of Advanced Nursing*
Visiting Professor of Nursing Studies
Bournemouth University

OXFORD
BLACKWELL SCIENTIFIC PUBLICATIONS
LONDON EDINBURGH BOSTON
MELBOURNE PARIS BERLIN VIENNA

This collection © 1994 by
Blackwell Scientific Publications
Editorial Offices:
Osney Mead, Oxford OX2 0EL
25 John Street, London WC1N 2BL
23 Ainslie Place, Edinburgh EH3 6AJ
238 Main Street, Cambridge,
    Massachusetts 02142, USA
54 University Street, Carlton,
    Victoria 3053, Australia

Other Editorial Offices:
Librairie Arnette SA
1, rue de Lille
75007 Paris
France

Blackwell Wissenschafts-Verlag GmbH
Düsseldorfer Str. 38
D-10707 Berlin
Germany

Blackwell MZV
Feldgasse 13
A-1238 Wien
Austria

This collection first published 1994
Full printing history of chapters can be found in the
Acknowledgements

Set by DP Photosetting, Aylesbury, Bucks
Printed and bound in Great Britain by
Hartnolls Ltd, Bodmin, Cornwall

DISTRIBUTORS
Marston Book Services Ltd
PO Box 87
Oxford OX2 0DT
(Orders: Tel: 0865 791155
         Fax: 0865 791927
         Telex: 837515)

USA
Blackwell Scientific Publications, Inc.
238 Main Street
Cambridge, MA 02142
(Orders: Tel: 800 759-6102
                617 876 7000)

Canada
Times Mirror Professional Publishing, Ltd
130 Flaska Drive
Markham, Ontario L6G 1B8
(Orders: Tel: 800 268-4178
               416 470-6739)

Australia
Blackwell Scientific Publications Pty Ltd
54 University Street
Carlton, Victoria 3053
(Orders: Tel: 03 347-5552)

British Library
Cataloguing in Publication Data
A Catalogue record for this book is available from
the British Library

ISBN 0–632–03865–9

Library of Congress
Cataloging in Publication Data
Models, theories, and concepts/edited by James
  P. Smith
        p.   cm.—(Advanced nursing series)
    Collection of updated papers originally
published in the Journal of advanced nursing
from 1989 to 1993.
    Includes bibliographical references and index.
    ISBN 0–632–03865–9
    1. Nursing—Philosophy.   2. Nursing
models.   I. Smith, James P.   II. Journal of
advanced nursing.   III. Series.
    [DNLM: 1. Nursing Theory—collected works.
2. Models, Nursing—collected works.
WY 86 M689 1994]
RT84.5.M64   1994
610.73′01—dc20
DNLM/DLC
for Library of Congress   93–49560
                                                CIP

Contents

List of contributors

Andrea Baumann, *RN, PhD*
Professor, School of Nursing, Faculty of Health Sciences, McMaster University, Hamilton, Ontario, Canada.

Ann C. Beckingham, *RN, PhD*
Professor, School of Nursing, Educational Centre for Aging and Health, McMaster University, Hamilton, Ontario, Canada.

Desmond F.S. Cormack, *RMN, RGN, MPhil, DipEd, DipN, PhD*
Honorary Reader in Health and Nursing, Queen Margaret College, Edinburgh, Scotland.

Carole A. Estabrooks, *MN, RN*
Doctoral Student, Faculty of Nursing, University of Alberta, Edmonton, Alberta, Canda.

Gordon Grant, *BSc, MSc, PhD*
Director, Centre for Social Policy Research and Development, University of Wales, Bangor, Gwynedd, Wales.

Rosemary Johnson, *PhD, RN, CS, NP*
Associate Professor, School of Nursing, University of Southern Maine, 96 Falmouth Street, Portland, Maine 04103, USA.

Janet B. Knight, *BScN, MScN, RN*
Assistant Professor, School of Nursing, University of Ottawa, Ottawa, Canada.

Marianne Lindell, *BSc (Nursing and Midwifery), UD in Nursing Education*
Doctoral Student/research assistant, Centre for Caring Sciences, Örebro, Sweden.

Kim Lützén, *Dr Med. Sc.*
Lecturer, Stockholm School of Health and Caring Sciences, Department of Nursing, and Doctoral Candidate, Department of Psychiatry, Karolinska Institute, Sweden.

Janice M. Morse, *PhD (Anthro), PhD (Nurs), RN*
Professor, School of Nursing, The Pennsylvania State University, University Park, Pennsylvania, USA.

Mike Nolan, *BEd, MA, MSc, PhD, RMN, RGN*
Senior Lecturer in Nursing Research, Health Studies Research Division, University of Wales, Bangor, Gwynedd, Wales.

Conny Nordin, *MD*
Associate Professor, Department of Psychiatry, Karolinska Institute, Huddinge University Hospital, Huddinge, Sweden.

Kerstin Hedberg Nyqvist, *RN, BSN*
Clinical Nurse Specialist, Neonatal Intensive Care Unit 95F, University Hospital, Uppsala, Sweden.

Henny Olsson, *PhD, BSc, BSc(Nursing, Midwifery and Public Health Nursing), UD in Nursing Education*
Professor pro tem, Research Supervisor, Center for Caring Sciences, Örebro Medical Center Hospital, Örebro, Sweden.

Mary Carol Ramos, *PhD, RN*
Quality Management Co-ordinator, Division of Health Care Evaluation, University of Virginia Hospital, Charlottesville, Virginia, USA.

William Reynolds, *RMN, RNT, RGN, MPhil*
Senior Tutor, Highland College of Nursing and Midwifery, Inverness, Scotland

Jane J.A. Robinson, *MA, PhD, MIPM, RGN, ONC, RHV, HVT*
Professor and Head of Department of Nursing and Midwifery Studies, University of Nottingham, Medical School, Queen's Medical Centre, Nottingham, England.

Beth, L. Rodgers, *PhD, RN*
Associate Professor, School of Nursing, University of Wisconsin-Milwaukee, Milwaukee, Wisconsin, USA.

Per-Olow Sjödén, *PhD*
Professor, Centre for Caring Sciences, Uppsala University, University Hospital, Uppsala, Sweden.

James P. Smith, *OBE, BSc (Soc), MSc, DER, SRN, RNT, BTA Certificate, FRCN, FRSH*
Editor of the *Journal of Advanced Nursing*, and Visiting Professor of Nursing Studies, Bournemouth University, England.

Sharon Williams Utz, *PhD, RN*
Associate Professor, School of Nursing, University of Virginia, Charlottesville, Virginia 22903, USA.

Introduction

JAMES P. SMITH

OBE, BSc (Soc), MSc, DER, SRN, RNT, BTA Certificate, FRCN, FRSH
Editor of the *Journal of Advanced Nursing*

A notion in the mind

A concept is nothing more than a notion formed in one's mind to help in a given situation. After further thought, refinement and/or research, a model may be derived which, following further work, may result in theory creation.

There may, of course, be constant and dynamic interplay between concept formation, model building and theory creation. Peers and academic supervisors will play an important role in that interplay. It is important, however, always to remember the important principle of refutation of any concept, model or theory. Furthermore, they should not be permitted to contaminate your mental hygiene insofar as they can militate against creative and lateral thinking.

They should never become unbreakable tablets of stone: the constant attempts of researchers to refute them and of scholars to challenge them must be constantly fostered and facilitated. However, in the final analysis, professional practitioners of nursing, midwifery and health visiting must use a mix of available knowledge, ability, judgement and intuition derived from professional experience when deciding to apply any concept, model or theory to their work. That is the right and responsibility of an autonomous, professional practitioner, which, I hasten to add, is very different from actions based on culpable ignorance.

This volume is the first in a new *Advanced Nursing Series* to help and inform undergraduate and postgraduate nursing students and their educators, and all practising nurses, midwives and health visitors and their managers. The book is based on a selection of twelve papers previously published in the *Journal of Advanced Nursing*. They are recent papers, having appeared in the journal in the past five years. Where appropriate, some authors have updated their papers for this publication.

A means of improving practice

In January 1976, at the launch of the *Journal of Advanced Nursing*, in my very first editorial I wrote that I hoped that the journal would become an international medium for the publication of nursing knowledge. I stressed that it was not intended that the journal should become an end in itself. Rather, that it must be a means towards the end of improving the effectiveness of the practice of nursing and midwifery. I want the new *Advanced Nursing Series* to have a similar goal.

The contents of this volume certainly reflect an international mix of scholarship. The authors, a group of aspiring and established scholars and researchers, come from Canada, England, Scotland, Sweden, USA and Wales. The contents of their chapters, which were chosen to provide the reader with a selection of concepts, models and theories, demonstrate that their scholarly pursuits have not been ends in themselves. They all focus on practice and much of what they write about and share is gleaned from studies in practice settings. The attempts to apply their work to the practice of nursing, midwifery and health visiting are both explicit and self-evident in their publications. What is more, and a very important aspect of their work, they constantly and critically evaluate their own and others' work. Assumptions are also identified.

It is noteworthy that a number of the authors also acknowledge and demonstrate the contribution of the work and literature of other disciplines to the development of nursing knowledge.

It is good to see reference made to commonly seen illnesses and health care problems, from contraceptive counselling by midwives to breastfeeding, mitral valve replacement, multiple sclerosis and weight loss. Attention is also given to touch, respite care for frail elderly people, the family in crisis, and hospital and community psychiatric care – all of which illustrate important functions in the nursing role: care, cure and prevention. The nursing problems discussed by the authors are real problems in the real world of nursing and health care of the 1990s. It is reassuring to note that scholars are devoting their energies to, and helping to create knowledge about, *practice* in nursing and health care.

What is also important is that the authors have identified important gaps in the state of knowledge. They also acknowledge deficiencies in some of the concepts, models and theories presently being used. Constant awareness of deficiencies will ensure that scholars and practitioners will guard against the danger of reifying these kinds of academic creations.

In fact, some of the authors have committed themselves to fairly long term follow up studies to re-evaluate their work and continue the search for 'truth' and a sound knowledge-base to narrow the often identified theory – practice gap. It is very reassuring that the nature of nursing knowledge and its relationship to practice have increasingly become key interests of scholars in recent years. It is particularly pleasing to note the serious and reflective consideration of the contributors in this book to concepts, models and theories, not as ends in themselves but as a means of enhancing the practice of nursing, midwifery and health visiting.

The state of nursing knowledge

Professor Robinson points out, in the first chapter, that it was her concern about the state of nursing knowledge and its relationship to health visiting practice which first stimulated her to embark on her own research in the 1970s. She was then (and remains) concerned about the absence of critical evaluation of the different theoretical perspectives taught to students and their influence on practice.

In her view, although nurses may apply natural science to their work, she argues that the activity of nursing is a social process. Therefore, she believes, the study of nursing and its understanding will involve the use of social investigation. Professor Robinson contends that some nurses have constrained the academic development of nursing by an inappropriate use of natural science terminology. She holds that the use of the term paradigm in relation to nursing is an inappropriate distraction. But, she adds, *thinking* about paradigms may be a useful intellectual exercise to bring order to a conceptual jumble.

Professor Robinson finally argues that:

> 'Ever increasing conceptual clarification in order to describe with rigour the social processes of nursing activity may not be sensational but it may be all that is available to us in our current state of knowledge development.'

Dr Rodgers takes as her starting point the current concern with the state of nursing's knowledge-base. She argues that the growing emphasis on concepts is appropriate as they promote the organization of experience, facilitate communication and 'enable the cognitive recall of phenomena that may not be immediately present'. But she wisely points out that when the definition or attributes of a concept are unclear, the concept's ability to assist in 'fundamental tasks' is greatly impaired.

Referring to the era of analytic philosophy and logical positivism and the academic traditions they fostered, Dr Rodgers points out that their tenets have now fallen into disrepute among contemporary philosophers. Yet, unfortunately, they persistently influence the current analyses in nursing. She shares some of her ideas about concept development that should overcome this state of affairs. She identifies a method of concept analysis which is simple, clear and uncomplicated, 'not imposing any strict criteria ... but simply seeing what is common in the existing use of the concept'.

Theory building

Dr Johnson discusses her analysis of the experience of dieters who attended a weight loss programme which she used to develop a substantive theory of restructuring. She identifies three stages. The first stage describes the need of the overweight person to be in charge of food. Stage 2 reflects the alteration in attitudes as the dieter loses weight. Stage 3 entails the dieter synthesizing former beliefs and habits into a new way of life. The three stages of the theory are illustrated in a model.

In the spirit of true and rigorous scholarship, Dr Johnson intends to continue testing her theory during a seven year follow-up study.

Focusing on hospital and community psychiatric care settings, Drs Lützén and Nordin describe how they developed the concept of benevolence from a grounded theory study of nursing decisions. In their view, benevolence is a central moral concept in psychiatric nursing as psychiatric nurses are often faced with making decisions on behalf of their patients. Therefore, they argue, the nurses 'wish to do good' on behalf of their patients. Their findings suggest that, if benevolence is an important attribute of psychiatric nurses, then there may be implications for the selection and placement of psychiatric nurses, particularly in what they call 'ungratifying' areas of clinical work. But perhaps others will want to challenge the right of psychiatric nurses to be making decisions on behalf of their patients at all!

Drs Nolan and Grant use a study of a respite care scheme for frail elderly people to build a mid-range theory, in an attempt to bridge the 'nursing theory–practice gap'. But, from the outset, they readily concede that the theoretical position of nursing is unclear; indeed, they consider it to be confusing. Because of this, they suggest that practitioners' reaction invariably results in them rejecting theory. It is this that causes the theory–practice gap, in their view.

They further claim that the use of theories and models in nursing has often resulted in sweeping generalizations which, they suggest, are not always appropriate – contextually, culturally or personally – to patients. They see mid-range theory building as more relevant to both patients and practitioners in the real world of practice. They do not see it as useful to search for a grand theory of nursing, given the diversity of nursing practice.

But, perhaps it is a question of patience and evolution, for Ms Estabrooks and Professor Morse, in their novel paper relating to touch, suggest that a conceptualization is an important stage in developing a theory of touch. Their work is based on a study in which they examined touch by nurses in an intensive care setting. An understanding of how nurses touch their patients clearly has implications for teachers of nursing. Ms Estabrooks and Professor Morse also illustrate how their work has contributed to theory development by adding to the existing work on touch.

That the activity of theory building can be particularly creative is demonstrated by the numbers of questions they pose for future investigations.

Neuman Systems Model and Roy Adaptation Model

The chapter by Ms Lindell and Professor Olsson is an interesting one, not only because of the topic – contraceptive counselling by Swedish midwives (who are responsible for up to 80% of the counselling) – but also for the conclusion. The authors conclude that the Neuman Systems Model can be used as a theoretical aid to facilitate contraceptive counselling by midwives, but they argue that it is not possible to predict how use of the model can increase the effectiveness of the birth control pill in preventing pregnancy and reducing the number of abortions. They advocate the need for further research.

The use of the Roy Adaptation Model as a conceptual structure for giving advice about breastfeeding to mothers of infants who are admitted to a neonatal intensive care unit is discussed by Ms Nyqvist and Professor Sjödén. Again, the attention is on a very important practical aspect of care. An important finding is that a modification of the model was deemed necessary. Namely, the incorporation of the 'interactive aspect of the attitudes, role functions and behaviour of nurses, and how they are perceived by patients and their families'. The authors also stress that the impact of theory on nursing needs to be tested further to establish its value to practical application.

Orem's Self-Care Deficit Theory

Orem's Self-Care Deficit Theory of Nursing is used by Drs Utz and Ramos as a theoretical framework for a number of completed studies of the nursing needs of patients with mitral valve prolapse. Whilst they found Orem's framework to be intuitively attractive, they decided that further clarification and empirical validation were necessary. (It is noteworthy that they concede the contribution of the medical literature in their work.) The four studies which they describe contribute a 'unique facet to the evolving research programme'. They also incorporated in their studies knowledge from other disciplines such as psychology and physiology.

Their final conclusion is worth reiterating:

> 'Although this approach may not be applicable to all nursing research, it is one method for promoting focused building of theoretical and clinical nursing knowledge.'

Ms Knight focuses on the care of a patient with multiple sclerosis. Her aim is to establish the 'goodness of fit' of the Neuman Systems Model. She believes that this model is ideally suited for guiding the nursing practice of a patient with multiple sclerosis. Her application to the care of a real patient is commendable and is a good role model for nursing students. Ms Knight's contribution illustrates the potentially exciting and satisfying nature of applying nursing models to practice. But as she notes, 'the variety of nursing phenomena and situations demands some flexibility in the choice of specific conceptualizations to be used'.

Integration of two models

The ageing family in crisis is the focus of the work of Drs Beckingham and Baumann. It is certainly a topic that will have a ring of reality for us all. The care of the ageing family is probably one of the greatest challenges facing all health care workers – and younger relatives – in the coming decades. The authors stress the importance of informed collaborative care: clients, families and health care workers alike. They have integrated the Calgary Family Assessment Model with the Neuman Systems Model to develop a comprehensive decision-making model.

The aim of their model is to guide health professionals in the identification of factors that may impede optimum decision-making. Their approach is praiseworthy and pragmatic. For, as they say, in the decision-making process related to health care, 'families must guard against paternalism ... In the long run, patients and families will do what they decide, not what we decide ...'. How very true – and rightly so.

Johnson Behavioural System Model

The final chapter, on the evaluation of the Johnson Behavioural System Model of Nursing by Mr Reynolds and Dr Cormack, is an excellent example of international collaboration. Data were collected in the USA; the authors live and work in Scotland.

As a starting point, they acknowledged that the model forms the basis of a primary nursing system and they set out to assess its relevance to clinical nursing practice. Fieldwork was carried out at the UCLA Neuropsychiatric Institute and Hospital, Los Angeles, USA. According to their criteria, the model was not entirely satisfactory and its clinical usefulness is considered to be limited by the authors. Nevertheless, they intend to continue to pursue this matter with tenacity and rigour. They also mention some ethical concerns about models.

Mr Reynolds and Dr Cormack point out that a number of nursing scholars consider nursing models to be pretentious, not least because nursing, being an applied science, borrows from other disciplines. But, they argue:

'What is important for the nursing profession is to know whether theory-based practice, irrespective of whether it comes from insights generated by nursing or from other disciplines, results in better care or improved health outcomes.'

I could not agree more.

Conclusion

By way of conclusion, I want to endorse some of the final comments made by Mr Reynolds and Dr Cormack in their chapter:

'Whilst the process of validating models would be facilitated if creators of nursing models addressed issues regarding practical and clinical utility, this process is also dependent on clinicians' clinical reasoning. This involves the ability to see things afresh and to be sensitive to the limits of existing information . . .'

That is surely a message for us all.

Chapter 1
Problems with paradigms in a caring profession

JANE J.A. ROBINSON, *MA, PhD, MIPM, RGN, ONC, RHV, HVT*

Professor and Head of Department of Nursing and Midwifery Studies, University of Nottingham, Medical School, Queen's Medical Centre, Nottingham, England

The terms 'paradigms' and 'paradigm shifts' entered everyday language following the publication in 1962 of Kuhn's book *The Structure of Scientific Revolutions*. Kuhn's original usage of these terms in relation to 'normal' science has since been inappropriately applied to other areas of formal knowledge. Their use in relation to nursing is conceptually flawed, and is an unnecessary distraction from the more modest, but nevertheless rigorous, approaches to the elucidation and generation of knowledge for practice which are required.

Epigraph

'... clearing intellectual jungles is (also) a respectable occupation. Perhaps every science must start with metaphor and end with algebra; and perhaps without the metaphor there would never have been any algebra.'

Max Black (1962)

Introduction

The nature of nursing knowledge and its relationship to practice (in my case, health visiting) were issues which concerned me greatly when I first embarked on research during the 1970s. Indeed, Chapter Two of *An Evaluation of Health Visiting* (Robinson, 1982), which is entitled 'Theoretical perspectives affecting the development of health visiting practice', concluded that:

'... the absence of any critical evaluation of the ways in which the different theoretical perspectives taught during ... training have influenced subsequent practice may have contributed to the role conflicts experienced by health visitors. The situation may have been exacerbated firstly by the assumption that integration of knowledge is both desirable and feasible, and secondly by the differing expectations of the health visitor held by various members of her role set.

It has been suggested that the health visitor may attempt to resolve the conflict inherent in certain situations by moving towards either a clinical or a social science perspective. Further exploration of this proposition would appear to be essential.'

Hopefully this statement establishes my personal credentials as a nurse who has long been deeply concerned with the relationship of knowledge to practice, as this paper embarks on a rather critical evaluation of some of nursing's more extreme claims to scientific knowledge. Colours should be nailed to the mast immediately and an admission made of extreme disquiet arising from some of the more extreme debates over the untested, hypothetical, highly abstract models of nursing which were taking place between 1985 and 1988. At the time, when acting as a temporary adviser to the World Health Organization European Region on the content and organization of a Conference on Nursing (held in Vienna in June 1988), a consultant joined us who had numerous models of nursing at her finger tips and these she exhorted us to adopt for European nursing practice (Robinson, 1987). A very small minority of these models did originate from Europe, but the vast majority emanated from North America where, as far as one was able to ascertain, they had rarely been tested empirically in the practice situation; the term 'empirical' to denote that '. . . the propositions of social science must be tested against observational data to survive as tenable generalisations . . .' (Bulmer, 1982).

It hardly needs pointing out how very different from Europe or the United Kingdom the health care culture is where the majority of the models had been developed. This call for general application without rigorous evaluation appeared therefore to be, at best, poor science; at worst it appeared to epitomize aspects of intellectual imperialism.

This is not to deny that a 'longing for a regular pattern into which the whole of human experience can be fitted' may be an extremely common phenomenon (Robinson, 1982). Olive Stevenson (who supervised both my higher degrees) has suggested that this longing for regularity in patterns of thinking is widespread. However, in the context of social work, she rejected the idea of a 'body of knowledge' as a prerequisite for social work's claim to professionalism, saying:

'To me . . . this phrase conveys an idea of something too static, too formed, to be possible or desirable in the present state of the social sciences and social work. It is vitally important that we should not be talking at this stage in our development as if the knowledge upon which we can draw had a shape and clear cut boundaries . . .'

Stevenson (1974)

Instead she developed the notion of 'frames of reference' which

> '... may complement or conflict. There is a pressing need to analyse these issues further and until this is done we will do little to help our students with the task of synthesis for practice which must be our ultimate objective. There must, for example, be rigorous comparative study of different approaches to the understanding of human behaviour so that we may see more clearly where there is genuine conflict, where merely semantic difficulties.'

Stevenson (1974)

There is much to commend this modest approach to the elucidation and generation of knowledge for practice to nursing, lest we all try to claim too much and end up looking ridiculous in the process. We shall be better academics if we recognize the multiple sources of knowledge on which we draw. Although we may apply *natural* science knowledge in some aspects of nursing practice (and therefore need to understand the different frames of reference to which natural science relates), we have also to distinguish between this knowledge and knowledge for the activities which we call 'nursing' and which in themselves represent a *social* process. This process has to be analysed with the tools which help us better to clarify and to develop the concepts which increase our understanding of what we call 'nursing' within it.

This aspect of nursing knowledge will be returned to later but, for the present, let us turn to 'paradigms and problems of a caring profession', which was the title originally given for this chapter. Although the title is interesting it is not clear what was intended in the context of nursing knowledge. It will be necessary therefore to *construct* what one believes *may* have been intended. This construction will attempt to show that, by using ambiguous and rather pretentious terms, nursing obscures rather than clarifies the conceptual foundations of its knowledge base. In carrying out this analysis it has become clear that the title as given was inappropriate. I have therefore presumed to alter it slightly but perhaps significantly to 'Problems with paradigms in a caring profession'.

Forms of knowledge: clearing the undergrowth

It is assumed that the term 'paradigm' refers loosely to Thomas Kuhn's usage in *The Structure of Scientific Revolutions* (Kuhn, 1962; 1970). Unfortunately, instead of helping, this focus reveals several problems relating to rigour and appropriateness which will be addressed in turn. First, Kuhn was a physicist who stumbled accidentally into the history of ideas surrounding his subject more than 10 years before he published the first edition of his account of scientific revolutions in 1962.

The impact of this book was undoubtedly startling. Regis (1987) asserts, for example, that

'... by 1968 Kuhn was one of the two or three most frequently cited authors in the United States. People suddenly began to see 'paradigms' and 'paradigm shifts' everywhere – almost as if it were a sport, an egghead recreation of some kind – and for a while your adroitness in juggling paradigmatic shifts and cosmic revolutions became an index of your meta-scientific enlightenment and degree of intellectual chic.'

Yet Kuhn's starting point was the study of the revolutionary phases in the development of *physics*. Central to his differentiation of the *natural* sciences was the idea of a 'paradigm'. On the one hand, he argues, lie 'mature' sciences with clearly established paradigms; on the other are those whose development is still at a pre-paradigmatic stage. Kuhn (1970) claims that the ability of key theorists

'... implicitly to define the legitimate problems and methods of a research field for succeeding generations of practitioners [lay in] two essential characteristics. Their achievement was sufficiently unprecedented to attract an enduring group of adherents away from competing modes of scientific activity. Simultaneously, it was sufficiently open-ended to leave all sorts of problems for the redefined group of practitioners to resolve.'

Kuhn continues (my emphasis):

'Achievements that share these two characteristics I shall henceforth refer to as "paradigms", a term that relates closely to "normal science". By choosing it, I mean to suggest that some accepted examples of actual scientific practice – examples which include law, theory, application and instrumentation together – provide *models* from which spring particular coherent traditions of scientific research.'

Kuhn asserts quite emphatically that an open question remains as to what parts of social science have yet acquired such paradigms at all (Kuhn, 1970). Here is the first problem. A major obstacle to the use of the term 'paradigm' in relation to nursing knowledge exists because, if the term is used as Kuhn describes it above, it can be seen to be quite inappropriate for nursing which is neither 'mature' nor 'normal' science.

An example of the imprecision which results from non-rigorous use of the terminology is shown in an article by Eriksson (1989) entitled 'Caring paradigms'. Citing a Swedish author, Törnebohm (1985), she claims that the paradigm consists of four components:

(1) The interests of the researcher/practitioner that describe what she *wants* to do.
(2) The competence of the researcher/practitioner sets that limits what she is *able* to do [sic].
(3) The world view of the researcher/practitioner consisting of a number of general assumptions about that part of reality in which she acts.
(4) The view of science which includes a comprehension of the development of the caring discipline, the present state of the research field, how the actual science is related to other sciences, what kind of issues the researchers in the field deal with, how they work, how the science is related to its territory and prospects of the development of the science in the future.

It is not necessary to lay claim to membership of a 'mature' or 'normal' scientific community in order to assert that this global view of nursing's world is unlikely to lead to acceptable scholarship but also that it will not facilitate the relationship of knowledge to practice.

The second problem with any attempt to extrapolate Kuhn's notion of paradigms to nursing lies in the critical distinction which has been made between the forms of knowledge with which we are concerned. Becher (1989), a philosopher, carried out ethnographic research in order to map 'the variegated territory of academic knowledge' and to explore 'the diverse characteristics of those who inhabit and cultivate it'. In a fascinating study of 220 academics in 12 different academic disciplines, Becher develops a taxonomy which applies to their knowledge forms and knowledge communities. The taxonomy includes distinctions between:

(1) Restricted/unrestricted knowledge.
(2) Hard/soft knowledge.
(3) Convergent/divergent communities.
(4) Pure/applied disciplines.

Physics emerges to the extreme left of the spectrum on all four dimensions. It is quantitative, has a well developed theoretical structure embracing causal propositions, generalizable findings and universal laws. Its community sense is convergent with a strong sense of commonality.

> '... collective kinship, a mutuality of interests, a shared intellectual style, a consensual understanding of 'profound simplicities', and even 'a quasi-religious belief in the unity of nature'. It is not easy to doubt that physicists share a particular way of approaching problems, a collective ideology and even a common world view.'

Becher (1989)

Nursing knowledge

It is not difficult to imagine from this analysis that any new developments which shook physicists' commonly-held world view would indeed constitute a 'revolution' in the Kuhnian sense of the word. To suggest that a similar perception may be held of nursing knowledge is frankly ludicrous for it has almost exactly opposite characteristics:

> '... unclear boundaries, problems which are broad in scope but loose in definition, a relatively unspecific theoretical structure, a concern with the qualitative and particular, and a reiterative pattern of enquiry.'
>
> Becher (1989)

Nurses resemble far more the geographers and pharmacists in Becher's study, being:

> ' "highly multidisciplinary", having numerous overlaps with neighbouring subject groups and a heterogeneous set of professional concerns. Papers in these two fields frequently appear in the journals of other disciplines, with the result that the journals dedicated to their own disciplines tend to be weakly supported and lacking in prestige.'

Nursing knowledge, furthermore, is like pharmacy in Becher's (1989) study: highly applied. Nursing's uncritical tendency to appropriate the methods and language of what it believes to be 'science' in an apparent attempt to appear 'scientific', without attempting to consider some of the related philosophical problems, is a matter of major concern. The term 'paradigm' does not, of course, appear too often in the nursing literature, but its synonym, 'model', in the sense of a pattern or exemplar, does.

In 1985, when I began to think a great deal about some nurses' claims to a unique 'nursing science', the literature was searched for a lead on a philosophy of science perspective on models. The search was not particularly fruitful although one text, Black's (1962) critique of the ways in which the term 'models' is used without rigour in natural scientific discourse, confirmed that impression abounds. If the critique is applicable to natural science, it is even more appropriate for nursing. Consider this introduction by McFarlane (1986) to the nature of nursing models:

> 'A great deal of the literature dealing with models is confusing, largely because the terminology is used inconsistently and the language is convoluted... As I write I have a number of models around me – an inkstand with a model of a 1918 field ambulance on it, a doll dressed as a Welsh lady, a platypus... A real black cat competes for space, but he is a cat; the model is a representation of him, as are all the other models representations only of the reality that they represent.

Models of nursing, then, are representations of the reality of nursing practice. They represent the factors at work and how they are related.'

Here is an example of what Black describes as the metaphorical: a descriptive term being transferred to some object to which it is not properly applicable. McFarlane here is mistakenly equating nursing models (whatever they may be) with models in the literal sense; that is, a three-dimensional miniature, 'more or less true to scale' (Black, 1962). Nurses may indeed use scale models, such as those of the heart or kidney, in order to learn about the structure and function of the human body, but these are emphatically *not* nursing models in the sense that McFarlane describes them.

Black (1962) goes on to discuss three further, distinct, types of model. The second, a type of design, something worthy of imitation – a model husband, model Ford or fashion model – are mentioned but then dismissed as irrelevant in Black's discussion. He then compares scale and analogue models, both of which are symbolic representations of some real or imaginary original. Scale models, however, rely upon visual identity. Analogue models, by contrast, are guided by the more abstract aim of reproducing the *structure* of the original inasmuch as there is a point-by-point correspondence between the model's pattern of relationships and the original. Black cites hydraulic models of economic systems or the use of electrical circuits in computers as examples of analogue models.

It is possible that nurses may use diagrams in their discussion of nursing models in the mistaken belief that they represent an analogue model. These diagrams may illustrate a hypothesized abstract relationship between certain elements in a health care system. Diagrams may play a useful role in helping nurses (especially novices) to conceptualize (say) the relationship between nursing, the person, the environment and health (overlapping circles are popular) but they are emphatically *not* analogue models: they are diagrams.

Mathematical models, Black's fourth example, involve the identification and mathematical manipulation of a number of relevant variables, selected either on the basis of common sense or derived from theoretical considerations. The models of nursing labour supply and wastage, or of a country's population growth, depending on certain assumptions, for example, about birth and death rates, are instances of mathematical models. There are inevitable drawbacks when they are applied – as nursing supply modelling illustrates – for the drastic simplification of a complex social reality can result in a risk of confusing the accuracy of the mathematics with the strength of empirical verification in the field. Nor can mathematics provide any *causal* explanation for the phenomena described; *strength of association* between two or more variables is the limit of the explanatory power of mathematical models.

From models to archetypes

If it has been suggested that nurses' aspirations to a form of nursing knowledge identified with the hard, pure, convergent and restricted sciences should be demolished; a way has been left open to discuss what is possible instead. Black's (1962) criticism of natural scientists' imprecise use of models does not leave them, or us, without a lifeline. Instead, he attempts to explain what some social scientists would call 'theorizing' but which he describes as the processes involved when there is 'an implicit or submerged model operating in a writer's thought'. Disliking the term 'metaphor' because of its inappropriate transfer to objects to which it is not properly applicable. Black substitutes the term 'conceptual archetype'. The following account mirrors some aspects of the grounded theorizing process which takes place when, as a qualitative social scientist studying nursing, I attempt to make conceptual connections and to build 'ideal types' of social reality from my empirical research observations:

> 'By an *archetype* I mean a systematic repertoire of ideas by means of which a given thinker describes, by *analogical extension*, some domain to which those ideas do not immediately and literally apply. Thus, a detailed account of a particular archetype would require a list of key words and expressions, with statements of their interconnection and paradigmatic meanings in the field from which they were originally drawn. This might then be supplemented by analysis of the ways in which the original meanings become extended in their analogical uses.'
>
> Black (1962)

I believe that the 'Black Hole Theory of Nursing' (which we applied humorously in the first instance to the phenomena that we observed in our study of nursing following the introduction of general management into the National Health Service) bears some relationship to the process of analogical extension which Black (1962) describes. It would not help in our analysis to call what is described in the following quotation a 'model', although an *analogy* can be seen between the balance of power of the physical forces which apparently maintain some form of equilibrium in the astronomical black hole, and the social forces which sustain nursing's invisibility in its social equivalent; forces which are, incidentally, imperfectly understood in either part of the analogy.

The following quotation describes the *process* of analogical extension in which we engaged during our research:

> 'Our "mulling over" of the meaning of our observations crystallised one day in that flash of insight which characterises the research enterprise and which we immediately labelled "The Black Hole Theory of Nursing". In

general, it appeared that I had been observing nurses many (but not all) of whom seemed defensively unable to see their work within a broad policy context. Philip Strong, on the other hand, had observed general managers and doctors who displayed the most profound ignorance about pressing nursing issues and practice. It appeared that even where nurses had become nationally known within nursing for taking their work forward in creative and imaginative ways, the local general managers and doctors could remain profoundly ignorant of such innovations. We suddenly realised that despite the impressive statistics (half a million workforce in the United Kingdom) nursing is relatively unimportant to government and to managers in comparison with medicine. It was *medicine* that the Griffiths reforms sought to control – *nursing* was merely caught in the crossfire! The tensions to which this situation gave rise – the nursing group locked into the gravitational force of its internal preoccupations, and the others, on the outside, unable or unwilling to look in and comprehend the nature of nursing's dilemmas – seemed to us to be the social equivalent of an astronomical Black Hole.'

Robinson et al. (1992)

From archetypes to conceptual analysis

Developing an analogy helps us to make the crucial distinction between 'as if' rather than 'as being' statements, and towards the end of his critique Black (1962) refers to what he describes as the existential use of models. If we use language appropriate to the model in thinking about the domain of its application we can work, according to Black's thesis, not *by* analogy but *through* analogy. Hence, considering the forces which help to hold nursing trapped in its invisibility has led me to think a great deal about the distribution of power and control both within and without the profession. Thinking in new ways is always painful and one's articulation of the issues feels crude and clumsy. Nevertheless, once one has begun to develop an argument around a particular 'frame of reference' it becomes much easier to marshal one's thoughts in coherent ways. Lukes' (1986) radical, three-dimensional view of power has helped me to see that one of the major forces which keeps nurses 'locked in' to the 'Black Hole' concerns 'the sheer weight of institutions' which serve to shape their cognitions, perceptions and preferences. As a result:

'. . . they accept their role in the existing order of things, either because they can see or imagine no alternative to it, or because they see it as natural and unchangeable, or because they value it as divinely ordained and beneficial. To assume that the absence of grievance equals genuine consensus is simply to rule out the possibility of false or manipulated consensus by definitial fiat.'

Lukes (1986)

Lukes' conceptual analysis to nursing policy issues has continued to be applied both in my own research and in a re-examination of other authors' work. In a recent chapter on 'Power, politics and policy analysis in nursing' (Robinson, 1991), thinking about Lukes' three-dimensional view of power helped in the development of a conceptual categorization of the empirical evidence contained in White's (1985, 1986, 1988) three volumes on *Political Issues in Nursing*. This following provisional categorization involved a great deal of painful conceptual development but, at the same time, yielded an extremely useful framework with which to begin to analyse the powerful tensions which exist within and without nursing:

'(1) Nursing as a force for challenge and change; the costs and benefits of unity.
(2) Contemporary health policy initiatives; the potential risks and benefits for nurses and their clients.
(3) The structure of nursing; its constraints and its potential for development.
(4) Class, gender and race in nursing.
(5) Nurses as oppressors and enablers; power for and against the client.'

Robinson (1991)

Knowledge is never static and in the chapter cited above an attempt is made to convey to readers both how isolating and how painful the process of conceptual development can be for the individual concerned, and also how tentative is the resultant framework. Nurses sometimes have an unfortunate tendency to seize on such analyses as though they are written in stone and not to see that subsequent challenge and reconceptualization is an essential part of knowledge generation. It is important, however, to recognize the ancestry of such ideas and to see how its genealogy can be traced, in the above case to Lukes' work and beyond.

Another simple, but extremely fruitful, framework for conceptual analysis of nursing issues was developed by Stacey (1976). It has helped me to classify nursing according to the conceptual dimensions of health which implicitly underpin different aspects of nursing practice. Stacey argues that health in Western society can be conceptualized along each of the three following dimensions:

(1) individual or collective;
(2) functional fitness or welfare (care);
(3) preventive, curative, ameliorative.

It does not take a very great leap of the imagination to see that the nurse who practises along the Individual Functional Fitness, Curative dimensions will hold a very different world view of nursing practice and health care intervention to one whose framework involves the Collective, Welfare, and Ameliorative dimensions. This analysis may help us to turn conflict between nurses into understanding – a process which is not helped by the pretentious and inappropriate use of the term 'paradigm'. What is required in the analysis is progressive conceptual clarification so that the various sources of knowledge on which nursing draws may be identified, together with their forms of application in the delivery of nursing care.

Conclusion: knowledge generation as a social process

In the introduction to this chapter it was asserted that, although we may *apply* the findings of natural science in our practice, the activity of nursing is a social process. Therefore, its study and understanding will involve the use of social investigations. Furthermore, some nurses, I would contend, have 'painted themselves into a corner' by their inappropriate appropriation of natural science terminology for the academic study of their activities. In a seminal paper on 'Concept and theory formation in the social sciences', Shutz (1962) helps to clarify many of the dilemmas which flow from what I believe may be described as a category mistake:

> '. . . authors are prevented from grasping the point of vital concern to social scientists by their basic philosophy of sensationalistic empiricism or logical positivism, which identifies experience with sensory observation and which assumes that the only alternative to controllable and, therefore, objective sensory observation is that of subjective and, therefore, uncontrollable and unverifiable introspection.'

Shutz continues:

> '(1) The primary goal of the social sciences is to obtain organised knowledge of social reality. By the term 'social reality' I wish to be understood the sum total of objects and occurrences within the social cultural world as experienced by the commonsense thinking of men living their daily lives among their fellow-men, connected with them in manifold relations of interaction. It is the world of cultural objects and social institutions in which we are all born, within which we have to find our bearings, and with which we have to come to terms. From the outset, we, the actors on the social scene, experience the world we live in as a world both of nature and of culture, not as a private but as an intersubjective one; that is, a world common to all of us, either actually given or potentially

accessible to everyone; and this involves intercommunication and language.

(2) All forms of naturalism and logical empiricism simply take for granted this social reality, which is the proper object of the social sciences. Inter-subjectivity, interaction, intercommunication and language are simply presupposed as the unclarified foundation of these theorists. They assume, as it were, that the social scientist has already solved his fundamental problem, before scientific enquiry starts.'

I have argued that the use of the term 'paradigm' in relation to nursing knowledge is an inappropriate distraction. Developed originally in order to contribute to a specific understanding of major theoretical shifts in physics, transfer of the term 'paradigm' to the unrestricted, divergent and applied forms of knowledge needed in nursing is not helpful. Nevertheless, *thinking* about paradigms may be a useful intellectual exercise, for that cognitive process has helped to bring order to my own long-standing conceptual jumble for this chapter.

Finally, however, it is necessary to return to the modest approach to the elucidation and generation of knowledge for practice advocated by Olive Stevenson (1974). Ever-increasing conceptual clarification in order to describe with rigour the social processes of nursing activity may not be sensational but it may be all that is available to us in our current stage of knowledge development. If this process helps us better to understand, explain and negotiate our way around the nursing and health care world then it is probably no mean achievement.

References

Becher, T. (1989) *Academic Tribes and Territories: Intellectual Enquiry and the Cultures of Disciplines*. The Society for Research into Higher Education. Open University Press, Milton Keynes.

Black, M. (1962) *Models and Metaphors*. University of Cornell Press, Ithaca.

Bulmer, M. (1982) *The Uses of Social Research, Social Investigation in Public Policy-Making*. Contemporary Social Research, No. 3, George, Allen and Unwin, London.

Eriksson, K. (1989) Caring paradigms. A study of the origins and the development of caring paradigms among nursing students. *Scandinavian Journal of Caring Sciences*, **3**(4), 169–76.

Kuhn, T. (1962, 1970) *The Structure of Scientific Revolutions*, 2nd edn. International Encyclopaedia of United Science, 2:2. The University of Chicago Press, Chicago.

Lukes, S. (1986) *Power: A Radical View*. Macmillan, London.

McFarlane, J. (1986) The value of models for care. in *Models for Nursing* (eds B. Kershaw & J. Salvage), pp. 1–6. John Wiley and Sons, Chichester.

Regis, E. (1987) *Who got Einstein's Office? Eccentricity and Genius at the Institute for Advanced Study*. Simon and Schuster, London.

Robinson, J. (1982) *An Evaluation of Health Visiting*. CETHV/ENB, London.

Robinson, J. (1987) Working towards the targets. *Senior Nurse*, **6**(3), 24–8.

Robinson, J. (1991). Power, politics and policy analysis in nursing. In *Nursing: A Knowledge Base for Practice* (eds A. Perry & M. Jolley), pp. 271–307. Edward Arnold, London.

Robinson, J., Gray, A., & Elkan, R. (1992) *Policy Issues in Nursing.* Open University Press, Milton Keynes.

Schutz, A. (1962) Concept and theory formation in the social sciences. Reprinted in *Sociological Theory and Philosophical Analysis* (1972) (eds D. Emmet & A. MacIntyre), pp. 1–19. Macmillan, London.

Stacey, M. (1976) *Concepts of health and illness: a working paper on the concepts and their relevance for research.* Paper produced for the Health and Health Policy Panel of the SSRC. University of Warwick (Mimeo), Coventry.

Stevenson, O. (1974) Knowledge for social work. *British Journal of Social Work,* 1(2), 225–37.

Törnebohm, H. (1985) Tutkijan maailmankuva ja strategia suomalaisissa hoitotieteen väitöskirjoissa-tieteenteoreettinen sisällönanalyysi. Oulun sairaanhoitooppilaitos, Tutkielma.

White, R. (1985, 1986, 1988) *Political Issues in Nursing.* John Wiley & Sons, Chichester.

Chapter 2
Concepts, analysis and the development of nursing knowledge: the evolutionary cycle

BETH L. RODGERS, *PhD, RN*

Associate Professor, School of Nursing, University of Wisconsin-Milwaukee, Milwaukee, Wisconsin, USA

Nursing currently evidences concern with the development and clarification of its knowledge base. As a part of this focus, attention has often been directed towards concepts and methods of clarification. Although the method of concept analysis has been employed often to provide conceptual clarity, the foundations and implications of conducting an analysis of a concept have not been well explored in nursing. In this chapter, the philosophical foundations of the approach to concept analysis popularized by Walker & Avant (1983) are examined. Modifications of this method are offered, along with a framework for interpreting the findings of an analysis. The result is a view of concepts and an approach to analysis that is rigorous and useful in the clarification of a variety of concepts of interest in nursing.

Introduction

In recent years, considerable attention has been directed towards the development and clarification of the knowledge base of nursing. A concern with concepts and the resolution of conceptual problems has increasingly emerged as a component of this process of intellectual advancement (Rodgers & Knafl 1993). Such an emphasis on concepts is appropriate, as concepts play an important role in the development of knowledge and even in the conduct of everyday existence. They promote the organization of experience, facilitate communication among individuals, and enable the cognitive recall of phenomena that may not be immediately present.

When the definition, or attributes, of a concept are not clear, the ability of the concept to assist in fundamental tasks is greatly impaired. In such situations it is difficult, at best, to identify an instance of a particular concept and to distinguish such an occurrence from one that is not an example of the concept. Similarly, it is difficult to differentiate between the concept of interest and other concepts that may be related. In other words, significant barriers are encountered in attempts to clearly label some event or phenomenon as an example of one concept. As a result, communication is impaired as questions regarding vague or ambiguous concepts are met with confused responses that are dependent upon individual and often *ad hoc* interpretations.

The method of concept analysis has been employed to bring about the desired degree of clarity for some concepts of interest (Boyd, 1985; Knafl & Deatrick, 1986; Rew, 1986; Walker & Avant, 1983). Indeed, the use of the method popularized in nursing by Chinn & Jacobs (1983), Chinn & Kramer (1991), and Walker & Avant (1983) has made a considerable contribution to nursing knowledge by attempting to clarify a variety of significant concepts.

However, the method of concept analysis has not been well understood in nursing. Most significant is the observation that nurse scholars who describe or employ the method have rarely explored the philosophical foundations and implications of conducting an analysis of a concept. As a result, it is not clear precisely how the method functions or how analysis of a concept actually contributes to further intellectual progression. While the availability of a clear conceptual definition has much appeal, the actual value of such a definition cannot be taken as self-evident. The continued productive use of the method of concept analysis thus warrants the exploration and critical examination of the philosophical foundations and implications of the method as it is currently employed in nursing.

Philosophical foundations of concept analysis

Discussion of the foundations of the currently popular approach to analysis requires an initial examination of philosophical traditions concerning concepts. Throughout epistemology, as in nursing, concepts have been at the centre of various debates regarding the nature of knowledge. In philosophy, this long history of discussion has given rise to two primary schools of thought, commonly referred to as the entity and dispositional views of concepts. Entity views generally regard a concept as some type of entity or 'thing', such as an abstract mental image or idea, a word with a specific grammatical function, an external unitary form, or an element in a system of formal logic. In contrast, dispositional views regard concepts as habits or abilities to perform certain behaviours, such as specific mental or physical acts or the capacity for word use. Entity views focus on the entity itself, regardless of the form of the concept, whereas dispositional views emphasize the use of concepts, the behaviours or capabilities that are possible as a result of an individual having a grasp of particular concepts.

These two views, both entity and dispositional, have persisted in various forms from the early classical period until the present time. The threads of entity theories may be traced through the works of such noted philosophers as Aristotle (1908), Frege (1970a), Kant (1965), Locke (1975), and in the early writings of Ludwig Wittgenstein (1981), to name a few, along with continuation of such thinking evidenced in the works of individuals generally associated with the logical positivism movement. Dispositional theories are less common in a pure form, but are best represented by the familiar works of Gilbert Ryle (1971a) and by the later writings of Wittgenstein (1968).

Analytic philosophy

The era of analytic philosophy and, particularly, the logical positivism movement, provide the foundation for the currently popular approach to analysis. Such an approach to analysis follows the entity view of concepts and can be seen in the method outlined by Walker & Avant (1983, 1988). Adhering to the tenet of positivism that rejects all metaphysical statements, the emphasis of analysis was placed on the physical aspect of concepts. The mental aspects of cognition were considered to be essentially inaccessible and, perhaps, even irrelevant for direct examination. As a result of this view, and based on a foundation provided by Descartes (1960), the world was seen as essentially divided into two realms – a realm of mental or private existence and a realm of physical or public experience (Rorty, 1979).

Analysis consequently became rather empirical in its orientation. Concepts were believed to be characterized by a rigid set of conditions both necessary and sufficient to identify an instance of the concept. They were to have clear and distinct boundaries if they were to be considered concepts at all (Frege, 1970b). Such views held that not only were there lines of division between concepts, but that concepts did not change over time, or even from this world to any other possible world. Concepts were considered to possess some inherent truth value, with the truth or falsity of a concept related to the extent to which the concept corresponded with an element, or with a possible element, of physical reality (Carnap, 1956; Frege, 1970a; Wittgenstein, 1981).

These underlying assumptions concerning necessary and sufficient conditions, rigid boundaries, and possible worlds, are evident in the approach that requires the investigator to construct borderline, contrary, illegitimate and invented cases as a part of the analysis (Chinn & Jacobs 1983; Smith & Medin 1981; Walker & Avant 1983, 1988). It values reduction in the attempt to isolate the apparent essence of a given concept rather than focusing on the vast interrelationships that exist in the world. Similarly, it presents a static view of the world, to the extent that concepts not only do not change through time but also remain constant across contexts. Such tenets have fallen into disrepute among contemporary philosophers with the demise of positivism and its emphasis on the value and context-free nature of knowledge and a focus on reduction. Yet such a foundation persists in the approach to analysis currently employed in nursing.

Adoption of a dispositional approach to analysis would surmount some of the difficulties associated with the predominant view. Particularly useful is the aspect of dispositional views that overcomes the distinction between the private and public realms of cognition by focusing on the use of concepts. Yet little direction concerning the method of analysis is available beyond this point. Most significant is the considerable amount of difficulty associated with the idea of 'use', as the term itself is vague or ambiguous. 'Use' may be considered as employment, or it may be regarded as common use or correct use. Noted British philosopher Gilbert Ryle (1971b) devoted a lengthy discussion to the question of 'use', and was able only to define it as 'a way of operating with something'. While this definition of use implies the existence of some context in which concepts and their use occur, there is no insight provided into what such a context might be.

An approach to concepts and analysis that overcomes difficulties with a positivistic or reductionistic view and that addresses contemporary concerns valuing dynamism and interrelationships within reality has not been available in nursing. As a result, efforts to clarify the conceptual foundation of nursing are subject to a variety of epistemic problems. However, an alternative view is available that seems to resolve many of the persistent difficulties and that may be of greater utility in nursing. Although a satisfactory approach cannot be found in the works of any one philosopher, the integration of views expressed by H.H. Price (1953), Richard Rorty (1979), Stephen Toulmin (1972), and those provided in the later writings of Ludwig Wittgenstein (1968), contribute greatly to an enhanced understanding of concepts. Such an approach has been described in detail by Rodgers (1989, 1993) and is referred to as the evolutionary view.

The evolutionary view of concepts

In the evolutionary view, a concept is considered to be an abstraction that is expressed in some form, either discursive or non-discursive. Through socialization and repeated public interaction, a concept becomes associated with a particular set of attributes that constitute the definition of the concept. Concepts are publicly manifested through certain behaviours, with linguistic behaviours being one significant form of manifestation. Concepts, therefore, are generally expressed in statements that indicate what are considered to be the attributes.

Concepts contribute to the continuing development of knowledge even outside the context of an existing theory through their explanatory or descriptive powers. When the attributes of a concept are unclear, the contribution made by the concept in this regard is greatly limited. Analysis of the common use of a concept enables it to be defined and, consequently, clarified. As a result, the concept may be used more effectively; its strengths and limitations may be evaluated and variations introduced that enhance the contribution the concept makes to the attainment of intellectual goals. Concepts, therefore, are continually subject to change. Rather than being characterized by fixed sets of necessary and sufficient conditions, and identified by appeal to strict rules of correspondence, the attributes of a concept appear as a cluster; situations or phenomena that are encountered are evaluated in reference to their resemblance, rather than strict correspondence, to the defined concept (Rodgers, 1989; Toulmin, 1972; Wittgenstein, 1968).

The cycle of concept development

This view of concepts may be further clarified by directing attention to the process of concept development. This process is illustrated as a cycle that continually progresses through time, as shown in Fig. 2.1. Three distinct influences on concept development are apparent: significance, use, and application. The significance of an existing concept plays an important role in the concept's continuing development. Toulmin (1972) points out that 'concepts acquire a meaning through serving the relevant human purpose in actual practical cases'. This 'relevant human purpose' is related to the concept's ability to assist in the resolution of problems, its ability to characterize phenomena adequately, thus furthering efforts towards

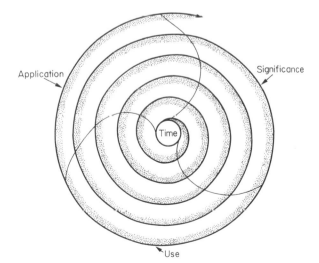

Fig. 2.1 Cycle of concept development.

achievement of intellectual ideals. As Toulmin indicates, significance is influenced by a variety of internal and external factors that provide incentives for the use and refinement of certain concepts to stimulate continuing development. A concept that is considered significant will be used often, ultimately facilitating the development of productive innovations and variations.

The significance of a concept thus has considerable impact on this frequency and extent of its use. The use of a concept, in this regard, is the common manner in which the concept is currently employed, the situations appropriate to its application, and whether or not the use occurs through language or some other form of presentation. Use carries with it the attributes of the concept that aid in the organization of human existence.

Application

As a concept becomes associated with a particular use, and this understanding is passed on through social interaction and education, there are continuing efforts to apply the concept in future encounters. Application thus results in the identification of the scope or range over which the concept is effective. Through the process of application, an existing concept may be continually refined, or conceptual variations and innovations may be introduced. As a result, the concept may be enhanced in its explanatory or descriptive powers, and may thereby offer a greater contribution to the attainment of intellectual ideals.

Over time, the use of a concept may become vague or ambiguous, or there may be concepts that appear to be in competition or conflict. Individuals who use a concept may be unable to articulate the attributes of the concept and the situations for its appropriate application, thus hindering efforts towards further knowledge development. Concept analysis aids in identifying the attributes of the concept through attention to its common use, thereby offering clarification and promoting efforts towards continuing development.

In this interpretation of concepts, the method of analysis is primarily a means of identification, not imposing any strict criteria, expectations, or view of reality on the concept, but simply seeing what is common in the existing use of the concept. The method involves a number of phases, rather than steps, as it does not proceed in a linear fashion (Rodgers, 1989, 1993). This revised method is shown in Table 2.1.

In contrast to traditional approaches to concept analysis, the identification or construction of borderline, contrary, invented and illegitimate cases is no longer considered to be appropriate. Such cases have been considered an important component of concept analysis based upon the assumption that concepts are characterized by a strict set of defining, or necessary and

Table 2.1   The method of concept analysis (evolutionary view).

---

(1) Identify the concept of interest and associated expressions.
(2) Identify and select an appropriate realm (sample) for data collection.
(3) Identify the attributes, references, antecedents, and consequences of the concept.
(4) Identify concepts that are related to the concept of interest.
(5) Conduct interdisciplinary, temporal, and other comparisons.
(6) Identify a model case of the concept, if appropriate.
(7) Identify implications for further development of the concept.

---

sufficient, conditions that do not change either over time or from one world to the next possible world. Such cases are not consistent with the view of concepts that underlies this revised method. Instead, their functions are addressed in the form of related concepts, a change that recognizes the interconnectedness of the world and the likelihood of change, rather than attempting to determine rigid lines of division.

Surrogate terms

When concept analysis is conducted in a linguistic manner, as it is most commonly employed, the identification of surrogate terms is an important step in the analysis. Individual concepts are not necessarily employed in association with only one specific term; rather, there may be several items which serve as manifestations of the concept. In addition, similar terms may be used to convey more than one concept, as is apparent in the number of homonyms evident in common language. Previously, such situations might have resulted in the identification of illegitimate cases of the concept. Such instances, however, more often refer to multiple unrelated uses of a term rather than to the inappropriate employment of a concept. A familiar example is that of 'coping', which has multiple uses including those pertaining to a type of architectural trim, a form of garment, and a type of wood cutting saw (Walker & Avant, 1983). Such examples cannot necessarily be considered as various, or perhaps illegitimate, uses of a particular concept, such as the concept regarding psychological or social alterations; rather, such instances are inherent in circumscribed language and are a problem of terminology rather than a problem of concept.

In this approach, attention is also directed towards the process of sample selection, an aspect of analysis that is not often adequately addressed. The means of sampling has a significant influence not only on the rigour of the analysis but on the findings as well. The use of a systematic means of sampling, such as selections drawn from computerized data bases, increases the likelihood that the items included in the analysis are representative of the total population (Guba & Lincoln, 1981), thus enhancing the credibility of the study. In addition, selection of a sample that includes items from various disciplines or domains enables examination of variations and similarities in the use of a concept across a broad field of concern. Finally, selection of a sample that addresses a broad time frame enables examination of the historical development or evolution of a concept and, consequently, of the continuing emergence of knowledge in a particular area of interest. Decisions regarding sampling techniques, therefore, may enhance the rigour of the study and contribute to the historical and contextual relevancy of the findings (Rodgers, 1993).

The model case has been retained as a significant aspect of concept analysis, although such cases are to be identified whenever possible, rather than constructed. A model case of a concept enhances the degree of clarification offered as a result of analysis by providing an everyday example that includes the attributes of the concept. The identification of references, antecedents and consequences has also been retained in this revised approach to concept analysis. The purpose of identifying the references of a concept is to clarify the range of events, situations, or phenomena over which the application of a concept is considered to be appropriate. The identification of antecedents and consequences provides further clarity regarding the concept of interest. The antecedents of a concept are the events or phenomena that are generally found to precede an instance of the concept; consequences follow an occurrence of the concept. Including these phases in the method of analysis provides additional information that may be useful in identifying what is an example of a particular concept and what is not-the-concept.

It is important to note that this method is not necessarily limited to linguistic applications. Certainly, the most common approach to concept analysis concerns an examination of literature items, and such a focus provides numerous benefits, not the least of which is related to the longevity of published items and institutionalization of language within a given social context. However, the method of concept analysis may be further developed to address concept use and application as they occur in non-discursive forms, such as the expression of concepts through physical behaviours or through the arts. Such an approach to inquiry may be beneficial in nursing and in the examination of various forms of communication and intervention.

Conclusion

Nursing has an interest in clarifying and developing its knowledge base and its conceptual foundation. The method of concept analysis offers a substantial contribution to continuing productive activity in this regard. However, it is a method with a complex and long-standing foundation in philosophy, a foundation and history that warrant consideration if the method is to be used effectively and to the benefits of nursing inquiry.

Recognizing the difficulties inherent in extant approaches to analysis and adopting subtle but significant changes in this method provides an approach that overcomes problems concerning the separation of the mental and physical realms of reality, that recognizes the dynamic and interrelated nature of the world, and that presents concepts as offering a pragmatic contribution to the resolution of existing and significant problems. While the resulting procedure may not be particularly new in philosophy, it presents a contemporary challenge to nurse researchers to re-evaluate the epistemic foundations and practical implications of existing approaches to concept analysis. Through further application and continuing evaluation of this approach, nursing may be able to develop a strong conceptual foundation to enhance efforts towards the continuing development of knowledge and the achievement of its goals throughout its domain of intellectual concern.

References

Aristotle (1908) *The Organon, or Logical Treatises with the Introduction of Porphyry*, Vol. 1–2 (trans. O.F. Owen). G. Bell, London.

Boyd, C. (1985) Toward an understanding of mother–daughter identification using concept analysis. *Advances in Nursing Science*, **7**(3), 78–86.

Carnap, R. (1956) *Meaning and Necessity*. University of Chicago Press, Chicago.

Chinn, P.L. & Jacobs, J.K. (1983) *Theory and Nursing: A Systematic Approach*. C.V. Mosby, St. Louis.

Chinn, P.L. & Kramer, M. (1991) *Theory and Nursing: A Systematic Approach*, 3rd edn. C.V. Mosby, St. Louis.

Descartes, R. (1960) Meditations on first philosophy. In *The European Philosophers from Descartes to Nietzsche* (ed. M.C. Beardsley). Modern Library, New York. (Original work published 1644).

Frege, G. (1970a) Function and concept (trans. P.T. Geach). In *Translations from the Philosophical Writings of Gottloh Frege* (eds P. Geach & M. Black) pp. 21–41. Basil Blackwell, Oxford. (Original work published 1952.)

Frege, G. (1970b) *Grundgesetze der Arithmetic* (Foundations of Arithmetic) (trans. P.T. Geach). In *Translations from the Philosophical Writings of Gottlob Frege* (eds P. Geach & M. Black) pp. 159–181. (Original work published 1952.)

Guba, E.G. & Lincoln, Y.S. (1981) *Effective Evaluation*. Jossey-Bass, San Francisco.

Kant, I. (1965) *Critique of Pure Reason* (trans. N.K. Smith). St Martin's Press, New York. (Original work published 1781.)

Knafl, K.A. & Deatrick, J.A. (1986) How families manage chronic conditions: an analysis of the concept of normalization. *Research in Nursing and Health*, **9**, 215–22.

Locke, J. (1975) *an Essay Concerning Human Understanding*. Oxford University Press, Oxford. (Original work published 1690.)

Price, H.H. (1953) *Thinking and Experience*. Hutchinson House, London.

Rew, L. (1986) Intuition: concept analysis of a group phenomenon. *Advances in Nursing Science*, **8**(2), 21–8.

Rodgers, B.L. (1989) The use and application of concepts in nursing: the case of health policy. (Doctoral dissertation, University of Virginia, 1987). *Dissertation Abstracts International*, **49**(11B) 4756.

Rodgers, B.L. (1993) Concept analysis: an evolutionary view. In *Concept Development in Nursing: Foundations, Techniques, and Application* (eds B.L. Rodgers & K.A. Knafl) pp. 73–92. W.B. Saunders, Philadelphia.

Rodgers, B.L. & Knafl, K.A. (eds) (1993) *Concept Development in Nursing: Foundations, Techniques, and Application.* W.B. Saunders, Philadelphia.

Rorty, R. (1979) *Philosophy and the Mirror of Nature.* Princeton University Press, Princeton.

Ryle, G. (1971a) Thinking thoughts and having concepts. In *Collected Papers* (Vol. 2) pp. 446–50. Hutchinson House, London.

Ryle, G. (1971b) Use, usage and meaning. In *Collected Papers* (Vol. 2) pp. 407–14. Hutchinson House, London.

Smith, E.E. & Medin, D.L. (1981) *Categories and Concepts.* Harvard University Press, Cambridge.

Toulmin, S. (1972) *Human Understanding.* Princeton University Press, Princeton.

Walker, L.O. & Avant, K.C. (1983) *Strategies for Theory Construction in Nursing.* Appleton–Century–Crofts, Norwalk, CT.

Walker, L.O. & Avant, K.C. (1988) *Strategies for Theory Construction in Nursing*, 2nd edn. Appleton & Lange, Norwalk, CT.

Wittgenstein, L. (1968) *Philosophical Investigations*, 3rd edn (trans. G.E.M. Anscombe). Macmillan, New York. (Original work published 1953.)

Wittgenstein, L. (1981) *Tractatus Logico-Philosophicus* (trans. D.F. Pears & B.F. McGuiness). Whitstable Litho, London. (Original work published 1921.)

Chapter 3
Restructuring: an emerging theory on the process of losing weight

ROSEMARY JOHNSON, *PhD, RN, CS, NP*
Associate Professor, School of Nursing, University of Southern Maine, 96 Falmouth Street, Portland, Maine 04103, USA

A qualitative research design (grounded theory) was used to analyse the experience of dieters attending a weight loss programme. Two hundred hours of observations at a nationally known weight reduction centre, a review of selected documents from the organization and multiple in-depth interviews with 13 informants were the data sources for this study. Data generation took place over a 21-month period. A substantive theory of restructuring identified three stages in the process of losing weight. These stages and key elements of the weight loss process are presented.

Introduction

The prevalence and seriousness of obesity and the high rate of relapse following treatment make it one of the most difficult health and psychological problems of our time. Cultural values in the United States also create tremendous social pressure to be thin. For the obese person, particularly women, this pressure often leads to an obsession with dieting (Chernin, 1981). Most individuals will lose weight; unfortunately, most will not remain thin. If 'cure' from obesity is defined as reduction to ideal weight and maintenance of that weight for five years, a person is more likely to recover from cancer than from obesity (VanItallie, 1979).

The literature abounds with research on the biologic, physiologic and psychosocial causes and effects of obesity (Bjorntorp, 1975; Dawber, 1980; Keesey, 1980; VanItallie, 1979), on predictors of successful weight loss (Colvin & Olson, 1983; Jeffrey *et al.*, 1984; Weiss, 1977) and on intervention strategies comparing and contrasting methods such as psychodynamic and behaviour modification (Stunkard & Mahoney, 1976; Wilson & Brownwell, 1980). Several authors have also discussed the importance of dominant and social cultural values about body size and aesthetics on weight maintenance (Allon, 1982; Rittenbaugh, 1982; Wooley & Wooley, 1984).

The subject of weight loss and maintenance has received little attention from nurse researchers. With few exceptions (Laffrey, 1986; Mallick, 1981), most nursing research has focused on a limited number of selected variables associated with obesity (Popkiss, 1981; Wineman, 1980). One promising area of nursing research examines *process* in relation to weight management. White (1984) identified five stages through which women progress as they enter treatment for obesity; Allan (1988) described the self-care practices of women managing their weight. The research described in this chapter begins where White's study ended and describes the informants' experiences while they work through the weight loss process, rather than a retrospective view of weight management strategies as presented in Allan's study. More studies are needed to address in depth the patterns and responses of dieters in the transition from overweight to a defined goal weight in order to facilitate the development of appropriate intervention strategies.

The purpose of this investigation was to generate data grounded in the conversations and observations of dieters undergoing the weight loss process. The goal was to understand their experience and develop substantive theory on the process of losing weight.

Methods

Setting

This study took place at a nationally known for-profit centre for weight reduction in the western part of the United States. Daily weigh-in and support is provided by counsellors who receive their training from personnel at the organization's headquarters. The typical profile of members in this programme is female, age 25 to 54 years, with an annual income of at least $20 000. The ratio of 10 women for every one man joining the programme is common, and no persons are under age 18.

Sample

The researcher informally interviewed and observed a number of dieters during fieldwork. From this mix of clients, 13 informants were chosen for in-depth interviewing. Theoretical sampling guided selection of these clients. With this sampling method, the researcher posed questions based on insights learned from coding data (Glaser & Strauss, 1967). This study group was white, well-educated, mainly professional women with a range of weight loss goals (18 to 122 pounds, $\bar{x} = 62$) and a variation in time of onset of the overweight problem.

Data generation

There were three sources of data in this study. First, the researchers observed 200 hours of weigh-ins, classes and seminars at the weight reduction centre. Second, multiple in-depth interviews were conducted with 13 informants, each lasting from 45 minutes to 2 hours over a 21-month period. Finally, all available documents relating to the setting were reviewed, including manuals, newsletters, magazines and informants' records.

Interviews were tape-recorded and both interviews and field notes from participant observations were transcribed. During the first interview, informants were asked to speak about their past history of being overweight to establish a context for their participation in a weight-loss programme. Initially, these interviews were unstructured. As more data were collected from both observations and interviews, informants' words were probed deeply for clarification, for broader descriptions of specific situations, and for the meaning behind some expressions.

Data analysis

The Ethnograph, a computer program developed by Seidel (1985), was utilized to assist in the mechanical aspects of data analysis. Data were coded and entered on the computer. Codes selected were words used by the informants or a word chosen to describe the major topic of discussion. These codes clustered to form categories. Categories were compared for relationships to each other, bringing key concepts into focus. Concepts such as control, perception, image/identity and support were generated. Once the main concepts emerged, additional data were collected for the specific purpose of elaborating the properties and variations of a category. This theoretical sampling process allows data to be collected to develop the theory (Glaser, 1978). Sampling continued until no new dimensions were generated, thus saturation of categories was reached (Glaser, 1978).

Following the identification of three stages in the process of losing weight, a literature review provided additional data to be woven into the analysis. The final step was to identify the process linking all the stages. Restructuring became that process link and formed the base of the emerging theory.

Credibility of the data

Grounded theory methodology comprises techniques to enhance the credibility of data. These are constant comparison of data, theoretical sampling and saturation of categories. Other measures to increase credibility in this study included extensive involvement at the site as a result of a lengthy data generation period and member checks at individual interviews, at group meetings and at the termination of the study. Researcher self-monitoring was accomplished by conversing with colleagues and dieters outside the study in order to gain their reaction to the investigator's thoughts on the emerging model. Triangulation of emerging data compared with professional and lay literature on the topics of weight management, transition and transformation also helped to increase the credibility of the findings.

The restructuring process identified in this study applied to those who remained in the programme as well as to those who left, since the researcher completed interviews on all informants regardless of whether they completed the organized programme or not. The sample also included people with varying weight-loss goals as well as those with the onset of a weight problem as a child, teenager and adult, further broadening the context of the findings. However, since the sample included predominantly white, well-educated, middle-class women, the findings are applicable to this group only until a different population is studied.

Restructuring

A basic social-psychological process called restructuring facilitates dieters' efforts to reach and maintain ideal weight. Restructuring represents the organization of and ongoing need for alteration of the dieter's life during and after the process of change from overweight to normal weight. An internal restructuring of self and external restructuring of the environment takes place. The restructuring which occurs at the start of the programme is more external in nature and does not require the same level of awareness necessary for the internal restructuring of self.

Depending on the phase within the process, internal and external restructuring may occur simultaneously or one form of restructuring may set the stage for the other. The strategies used by informants to manage their weight are viewed on a continuum from very rigid to very flexible. In this study, the degree of rigidity/flexibility varied, depending on past experience with success or failure.

Restructuring has three stages: gaining a sense of control, changing perspective and integrating a new identity and/or way of life. These stages of this basic social–psychological process are depicted in Fig. 3.1.

Stage 1: Gaining a sense of control

The first stage describes the need of the overweight person to be in charge of food. Both external and internal restructuring begin in stage 1. This first stage in the restructuring process takes time to achieve and involves many highs and lows for the individual before he or she can feel 'in control'. This

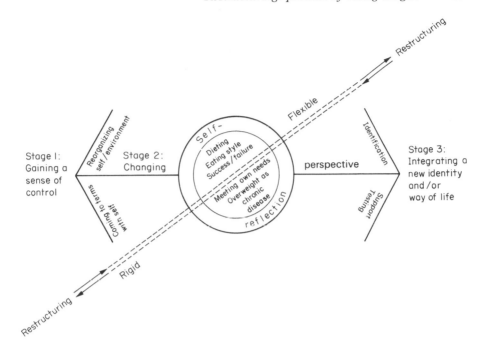

Fig. 3.1 Three stages of restructuring.

goal is accomplished in two phases, reorganizing self/environment and coming to terms with self.

During the *reorganizing self/environment* phase of gaining a sense of control, dieters utilized three strategies: seeking guidance or support by joining a weight reduction centre (programme monitoring); disciplining oneself through denial, either guided or self-imposed (keeping busy, avoiding social eating events); and creating a supportive environment. These three strategies are discussed by informants in the following excerpts:

> 'I realized that if I didn't get some very instructive help I would have this thing on my back.
>
> I used to eat out a lot but I don't do that any more . . . I just cook at home.
>
> I'm getting all of the things out of the way that I could use for an excuse. I'm not even watching TV very much . . . TV is loaded with commercials about eating all the wrong things . . . I've tried to surround myself with things that are going to be positive.'

The need for guidance and the desire to 'not go it alone' were common to all of the dieters. Self-denial, coupled with avoidance strategies, dominated the early phase of weight loss. In this first stage, most dieters found comfort and relief with the 'simplicity' of the routine and did not view restructuring as deprivation. The ability to relax and not become obsessed about food allowed for the time and energy to begin looking inward and to prepare to deal with the role of overeating. This brought the dieter to the second phase in the process of gaining a sense of control: coming to terms with self.

Coming to terms with self is a reflective period when the person has internal dialogue and accepts responsibility for making a major change in lifestyle. This is accomplished by a three-step process. Awareness of the role of overeating is the first step. One young woman who developed a problem with weight in her teens and had been married for two years stated:

> 'I always felt like my weight was a barrier to intimacy. I consistently sneaked food . . . I wasn't letting him get close to me. I was keeping kind of a layer away. I guess it takes a while to trust somebody – and so, it feels like by losing some weight I've gotten a little closer to him.'

This dieter used overweight to avoid intimacy and protect herself from being hurt. Understanding the function of food is critical to developing alternative ways of fulfilling needs previously met by food.

Awareness of alternatives leads to the second step in the process, realizing choices can and must be made. Once alternatives surface, there is a capability for choice: the dieter may either continue to function in his or her former way or break out of that mould. The third step, making up the mind and taking action, pertains to following through on the chosen alternatives. One informant captured the latter two steps in coming to terms with self when she stated:

> 'I made up my mind . . . I was going to do something for myself. I cut my hair, pierced my ears, and started on a diet . . . We are responsible for our own attitudes and spirit and can feel in control.'

Overlap does occur in the phases of the process in stage 1. However, the external restructuring taking place with reorganizing self/environment facilitated the internal restructuring with awareness in coming to terms with self. Coming to terms with self increased the degrees of self-trust which tempered the need for rigid restructuring. The time it took to gain a sense of control was influenced by the length of time the person had been overweight, by whether or not the function served by food was psychological or situational in origin, and also by the changing perspective of the dieter, which is the second stage in the dieter's restructuring process.

Stage 2: Changing perspective

Stage 2 reflects the alteration in attitude and outlook as the dieters continue to work through the process of losing weight. It is the thought process which begins with awareness in coming to terms with self. Changing perspective bridges the other two stages and is central to the entire restructuring process.

This changing level of awareness involves an internal restructuring of self which may affect the dieter's relationship with others, necessitating further restructuring of her social and physical environment. Without this change in perspective, the weight reducing plan is merely a programme to complete in order to reach a desired weight, rather than the beginning of a new approach to food, eating and lifestyle.

The key to changing perspective was self-reflection. Patterns emerged across informants on the themes for self-reflection. These included: meeting one's own needs, the meaning of success and failure, eating style and dieting, and overweight as a chronic disease.

Meeting one's own needs surfaced as an important priority. Having reached an awareness in stage 1 that food served a function beyond physical nourishment, the notion of 'hunger' as metaphor began to have deeper meaning during stage 2. This realization, that 'hunger' is not as simple as acquiring thinness and changing the shape of one's body, begins the process of changing perspective on how to achieve and maintain a desirable weight.

The majority of dieters in this study were women. Historically, women have been considered the primary caregivers, although the stereotype is changing. Pressures to conform to this stereotype caused women in this study to put the needs of others before their own. Some extremely overweight individuals felt the need to be overly nice to others in order to compensate for obesity which they viewed as a major handicap to relationships. As the dieters became more aware of these tendencies, they began to rethink and reorder priorities in their relationships with others. One woman spoke of this changing perspective.

> 'She admitted to using me and taking advantage of me. Probably if I hadn't gone through this process of finding out more about myself, I would have said, Oh wow, she needs me! ... If people think my friendships are based upon my being needed, then this is not their fault, it's mine!'

At this point the dieter began to view her needs as important. There was less guilt associated with not meeting the needs of others first. A theme of assertiveness was common. Emotions such as anger and fear that frequently precipitated eating for some informants were redirected through a strategy of being assertive. Assertiveness provided the person with another way to meet her own needs for nourishment in a constructive manner.

Relabelling the meaning of *success and failure* was another issue for change. The dieters became very upset with themselves when they overate. Overeating precipitated further eating. A change in perspective occurred as the dieter reconsidered how to respond to occasional overeating and a weight gain. In the second stage of restructuring, dieters changed their perception of what constituted success or failure. Singular episodes of overeating were no longer labelled failure. A dieter who spoke of living in extremes, i.e. either overeating or dieting, talked about realizing this perspective:

> 'There are times when it is alright to gain a few pounds. You are probably going to gain 2 to 5 pounds on vacation. That is okay, that is life. If you are going to go out and party and drink and eat pizza tonight that does not mean for the next few days you have to eat pizza.'

This change in perspective effected an increased sense of responsibility. The dieters realized he or she could be instrumental in dealing with certain food temptations by changing behaviour. This action brought with it a sense of control.

Uncovering the origins of *eating style and dieting* was frequently discussed. Informants talked about childhood habits and how these habits had been maintained. Reflection on the past helped them to view their present situation in a new light. One woman discussed the competitive nature of mealtimes in her childhood home. She ate fast and as much as she could in order not to go away hungry. She spoke of her efforts to change former habits:

> 'What I try to do now at mealtime is cook and serve only what we can eat ... there are no leftovers ... I've tried to get away from family-style cooking – eat all you want. We don't need that quantity.'

The process of changing perspective extended beyond weight loss. It broadened the view of weight management and was key to weight control. As one woman stated:

> 'I have to change, not just get down to my goal weight, but change my lifestyle in some way that I will be different and not go back to the same old habits.'

These new perspectives were the impetus for change in both eating style and dieting.

Recognizing *overweight as a chronic disease* was often discussed as being analogous with alcoholism, particularly among those who were compulsive eaters. The following comments are typical of informants:

> 'It's like being an alcoholic ... obesity is a disease. It is not curable but it is treatable.'

> ' "Bingeing" – my old friend. I may do it on occasion for the rest of my life ... It is a compulsive behaviour, like drinking leading to alcoholism for some people. It is something I will always have to deal with.'

A variety of skills can be adopted to maintain a thin exterior but the dieter must continue to be a controlled eater whose maintenance depends on vigilance. This changing perspective was gradual but viewed as critical to maintenance of weight loss.

The attitude and revelation expressed by the dieters in this study reinforces Adler's concept of lifestyle change (Ansbacher & Ansbacher, 1956). As each dieter developed a greater awareness of self, through the process of coming to terms with self, then changing perspective for 'permanent relief' from being overweight was brought into focus. This enhanced the creative possibilities for change. Desire for permanent relief from the overweight concern necessitated a commitment to integrating a new identity and/or way of life for the dieter – the third stage in the process of losing weight.

Stage 3: Integrating a new identity and/or way of life

In this last stage, meanings, values and behaviour patterns developed in the first two stages of the weight loss process are synthesized with former beliefs and habits. Testing, identification and support are important phases of this stage.

Testing entails finding the limit of one's food intake. By trial and error approaches, the former dieter learns his or her capabilities in handling food. Testing is frightening, but mastering this control brings with it a feeling of balance. During the testing period, there was movement away from denial and avoidance strategies (not allowing oneself the pleasures of certain foods or not eating out or not having company to dinner) toward distancing, discriminating and substituting. In this study, this included only eating ice cream outside the home (distancing) or choosing the 'best' chocolate if one must indulge (discriminating) or using less concentrated sweets to satisfy a craving (substituting), all intended to prevent bingeing.

Identification of oneself as a thin person is the major restructuring task of stage 3. During the weight-loss process, issues of body image and self-image arise, creating a mix of internal and external pressures for the dieter. A woman described a conflict which reflects a discrepancy between what she viewed as thin enough for her, and the ideal set by a thin-conscious society:

> 'When no one else is around I look in the mirror at myself – I look good. If someone else comes into the room, I look fat. I see myself differently when someone else is around.'

As the desired weight is achieved and maintained, the dieter begins consolidating his or her identity and new way of living as a thin person. These changes involve resolving any conflicts about the meaning of being thin as opposed to being fat. Resolution of these conflicts involves a transition from a 'fat' to a 'thin' mentality. While conflicts are more likely to exist for those who have been overweight since childhood, the adult person who has been overweight for a long time also needs more time to adapt to the thin image. A steady gradual weight loss rather than quick-reducing diets accommodated this need, as expressed by a woman who was 70 pounds overweight for much of her adult life.

> 'I think it's been good for me because I've adjusted better to my new self, and my friends certainly have ... I think that was my problem on previous diets. I lost too quick, to a point where I could see a change in myself; it got scary. You ask, who is that person? It has been so long and how will you handle it.'

Developing a 'thin' mentality may not be as difficult for the adult who has recently become overweight. However, to maintain weight loss, both types of overweight individuals must fully integrate a new way of eating and living. They must accept ongoing limits on food intake and an exercise regimen as a daily activity.

Support from family and friends facilitated the integration of a thin identity and lifestyle. Effective and tangible support were considered most helpful. This support was reported as a willingness to share some of the same meals, exercising together, and occasional complementary feedback on success of appearance. The amount of support that was needed varied with each person, based on her affiliation need. What was crucial was that significant others did not sabotage efforts. Examples cited were: leaving left-over or half-eaten snacks around the house, a mother-in-law sending homemade cookies to the house though aware that the entire family was dieting, or the well-intentioned, nagging reminders of what the dieter should and should not eat. This behaviour was easier to cope with as the dieter's self-reliance increased and she gained confidence in her ability to deal with a new lifestyle. As the structure initially imposed by the diet organization decreases, it must be emphasized that supportive structures developed during reducing continue to be important, particularly during maintenance.

In working through the three stages of the weight-loss process, informants found their ongoing struggle tempered by a new freedom and sense of self-worth as weight was maintained. The comments of two women are typical of others in this study:

> 'I feel a freedom to not worry ... about my rear as I walk away from people.'

> 'I finally care about myself.'

Discussion

This study identified a three-stage process called restructuring through which dieters progressed as they attempted to lose and maintain a goal weight. The process occurred over a period of time and involved change. While informants experienced the stages of the process in a step-wise fashion, parts of these stages may also be experienced simultaneously, and backsliding to previous stages may occur.

Maintaining weight loss by restructuring one's internal and external environment is a complex process. It reflects the relationship of the major concepts of significance – control, perception and identity/image. In the theoretical model of restructuring, behavioural and cognitive strategies are the means dieters utilized to achieve transformation. These concepts are not new; however, using them to discuss overweight from a process viewpoint is new.

The usual definitions used to operationalize the concept of control have been guided by a static view of control (Langer, 1983). Langer believes that these definitions 'rely primarily on outcomes rather than on the process of achieving those outcomes' and outcomes are assumed to be positive or negative. She reminds us that, in reality, outcomes are positive with respect to some standards and negative with respect to others. In the theoretical model of restructuring, control is viewed as an ongoing process as the dieter develops competence and skill in dealing with both internal and external environments. Consistent with Langer's (1983) view on process, 'one should pay attention to the way responses are exercised' and not to outcome alone.

Perception

Perception, the underlying concept of stage 2 (changing perspective), is pivotal to the restructuring process. In this stage, dieters identified four themes which affected their ability to gain a sense of control and integrate a new identity and/or way of life – the first and last stages of the weight-loss process. To facilitate this process, reflective strategies used included keeping a diary, lengthy walks alone and writing a novel. Regular use of these strategies gave meaning to each individual effort and personalized the solution to each weight problem. The reshaping of views accomplished in changing perspective is similar to the process of cognitive restructuring described by Beck (1976) as a therapeutic intervention in psychotherapy. The perceptual process occurring in both instances is cognitive reappraisal of views as conceptualized by Lazarus & Folkman (1984). With the dieters in this study, however, this was an intuitive process as opposed to a formalized, structured method.

A continual shift in perception and outlook resulted in a discarding of old views and habits. No single factor guaranteed the transformation but a series of events occurring over time, when completed, assured the individual of his or her identity as a thin person. Identification of oneself as a thin person is a major component of stage 3 in the restructuring model.

During testing in stage 2, the first marker of establishing a new identity is the ability to resist the temptation of certain foods that are taboo. When these 'taboo foods' ceased to tempt, when past favourite foods had lost their magnetic appeal and the craving was gone, then the transformation was further reinforced. The ability to monitor oneself without having to rely on the counsellor was also a marker that the person had internalized the values of her role model. These experiences are the hallmark that reinforce reality. In this study, these scenarios were common to those who had more weight to lose and who had followed a weight control regimen for a longer period. Nonetheless, all had to work through the testing phase. This proposition is consistent with Strauss's (1969) work on the search for identity when he states 'all persons deliberately court temptation as a form of self-test' to judge whether the transformation is complete.

Biological correlates

The stages of restructuring which emerged in this study emphasized the psychosocial dynamics of the transformation. This does not deny the fact that there are biological correlates which may affect the degree of difficulty in maintaining weight loss. Since a person's being encompasses the psychosocial and physiologic, both areas must be considered in order to deal adequately with the subject of being overweight. Knowledge of the biochemical and genetic theories will enable us to understand what worsens or improves the risk factors and will give credence to why some must work harder in monitoring their weight. Response to the application of this knowledge is part of the dynamics of the process identified in this study.

Implications

The findings of this study have important implications for the nurse working with clients, particularly women, who are struggling with trying to lose weight and maintain the loss. Progression through the three stages of the weight-loss process varied according to how well the individual could master the four themes of concern in changing perspective. In a clinical setting, nurses might aid in facilitating this process by incorporating cognitive strategies for intervention, rather than relying on behavioural techniques as is frequently the case. The use of cognitive strategies has been advocated by feminists for women with a weight concern (Orbach, 1978; Chernin, 1981; Roth, 1982) but it is not a common approach within the health care system.

The stories of dieters in this study emphasized that daily social pressures include contradictory messages that create obstacles to achieving the desired weight. The pressure to be thin also causes many to follow fad diets and encourages others, who are only 10 to 20% overweight, to continually diet. In trying to maintain an 'ideal' weight, some individuals may be inducing psychological strain more harmful to health and quality of life than the consequence of additional pounds.

Consciousness raising

It is important that nurses take a critical look at the social and cultural implications of being overweight and how it affects the care they offer to clients. The meaning of success and failure in weight loss must include parameters beyond scale weight. It will be viewed in this manner only if we think of weight loss as a process rather than an outcome. Nurses need to raise their own consciousness and that of their clients on this subject.

Further research of the stages developed in this study, utilizing both men and women with differing ethnic and socio-economic backgrounds, will help to broaden the usefulness of the model. This model could be studied for its application to transforming processes in other lifestyle changes such as abusive to non-abusive drinker or smoker to non-smoker. An umbrella model could then be formulated and applied to all transforming processes but will be more detailed in explaining the contexts and contingencies for specific change conditions. The testing of processes discovered in one substantive area (weight loss) with other conditions (alcohol abuse, smoking) would raise the level of the substantive theory on weight loss to that of a formal theory (Glaser & Strauss, 1967) about change or transformation.

Latest research activity

Since publication of Johnson's (1990) research, review of the literature has identified two pieces of research work (Prochaska *et al.*, 1992a; Allan, 1991), both with differing research programmes, yet their findings and interpretations are relevant to the area of weight management. For about twenty years, Prochaska and colleagues had refined and tested their model on behaviours such as psychological distress and smoking, and only recently was the model applied to weight management.

Prochaska using a quantitative design applied transtheoretical constructs of stages and processes of change to predict success in weight control (Prochaska *et al.*, 1992b); while Allan (1991), like Johnson, used a qualitative design to describe a weight loss process. In spite of the different research methods used to develop the models in the three studies, strikingly similar concepts were addressed, though language and interpretations differ based on the underlying assumptions of the two approaches used.

Process variables identified by Prochaska *et al.*, (1992b) included those cognitive and behavioural strategies also described by participants in both Allan's (1991) and Johnson's (1990) studies. Consciousness raising and self-evaluation – two change process variables in Prochaska's work – are also processes synonymous with changing perspective in Johnson's model.

Of interest is that Prochaska found that prolongation of these two processes was a deterrent to moving towards action strategies for weight management. His writing implies this to be a negative, since it delays weight loss. This seems inconsistent with a process model, since it infers the stages are time bound; Johnson's process was not time bound. An underlying assumption of Prochaska's work is that completion of the programme is positive. Johnson interviewed persons who completed as well as quit a programme. It was those individuals who were able to identify personalized solutions to their weight who were viewed as successful, whether or not they completed the programme. Allan (1991) also speaks of the importance of personalized solutions to weight management.

Prochaska's goal is to identify critical times for strategic interventions using change processes. This would be useful to health care providers, including nurses. However, in applying this knowledge, Johnson (1990) continues to advocate that markers of success should move beyond scale weight. This would be consistent with Prochaska's shift from a linear to a spiral process of change in weight management.

Seven year follow-up

Uncovering research on weight management that incorporates a process approach is most encouraging and should help in the identification of intervention strategies to assist clients with weight management. The literature cited complements Johnson's work but would not change her model. A seven year follow-up investigation of her theoretical model of restructuring will study the suitability of the model for weight maintenance.

Acknowledgements

This study was supported by a National Research Service Award (number NU-05701-02) from the National Institutes of Health, Bethesda, Maryland, USA.

References

Allan, J. (1988) Knowing what to weigh: women's self-care activities related to weight. *Advances in Nursing Science*, **11**(1), 47–60.

Allan, J.D. (1991) To lose, to maintain, to ignore: weight management among women. *Health Care for Women International*, **12**(2), 223–35.

Allon, N. (1982) The stigma of obesity in everyday life. In *Psychological Aspects of Obesity* (ed. B. Wolman) pp. 130–74. Van Nostrand, New York.

Ansbacher, H. & Ansbacher, R. (1956) *The Individual Psychology of Alfred Adler*. Harper & Row, New York.

Beck, A.T. (1976) *Cognitive Therapy and the Emotional Disorders*. New American Library, New York.

Bjorntorp, P. (1975) Effect of energy-reducing dietary regimen in relation to adipose tissue cellularity in obese women. *American Journal of Nutrition*, **28**, 445–52.

Chernin, K. (1981) *The Obsession: Reflection on the Tyranny of Slenderness*. Harper & Row, New York.

Colvin, R.H. & Olson, S. (1983) A descriptive analysis of men and women who have lost significant weight and are highly successful at maintaining the loss. *Addictive Behaviors*, **8**, 287–94.

Dawber, T.R. (1980) *The Framingham Study: The Epidemiology of Atherosclerotic Disease*. Harvard University Press, Cambridge.

Glaser, B.G. (1978) *Theoretical Sensitivity*. Sociology Press, San Francisco.

Glaser, B.G. & Strauss, A.L. (1967) *The Discovery of Grounded Theory: Strategies for Qualitative Research*. Aldine, New York.

Jeffrey, R.W., Bjorn-Benson, M.W., Rosenthal, B.S., Lindquist, R.A., Kurth, C.L. & Johnson, S.L. (1984) Correlates of weight loss and its maintenance over two years of follow-up among middle-aged men. *Preventive Medicine*, **13**, 155–68.

Johnson, R. (1990) Restructuring: an emerging theory on the process of losing weight. *Journal of Advanced Nursing*, **15**, 1289–96.

Keesey, R.E. (1980) A set point analysis of the regulation of body weight. In *Obesity* (ed. A.J. Stunkard). pp. 144–165. W.B. Saunders, Philadelphia.

Laffrey, S. (1986) Normal and overweight adults: perceived weight and health behavior characteristics. *Nursing Research*, **35**(3), 173–7.

Langer, E. (1983) *The Psychology of Control*. Sage, California.

Lazarus, R. & Folkman, S. (1984) *Stress, Appraisal and Coping*. Springer, New York.

Mallick, M.J. (1981) The adverse effects of weight control in teenage girls. *Advances in Nursing Science*, **3**(2), 121–3.

Orbach, S. (1978) *Fat is a Feminist Issue*. Berkeley, California.

Popkiss, I. (1981) Assessment scales for determining the cognitive behavioral repertoire of the obese subject. *Western Journal of Nursing Research*, **3**(2), 199–215.

Prochaska, J.O., DiClemente, C.C., & Norcross, J.C. (1992a) In search of how people change: applications to addictive behaviors. *American Psychologist*, **47**(9), 1102–14.

Prochaska, J.O., Norcross, J.C., Fowler, J.L., Follick, M.J. & Abrams, D.B. (1992b) Attendance and outcome in a work site weight control program: processes and stages of change as process and predictor variables. *Addictive Behaviors*, **17**(1), 35–45.

Rittenbaugh, C. (1982) Obesity as a culture-bound syndrome. *Culture, Medicine and Psychiatry*, **6**, 347–81.

Roth, G. (1982) *Feeding the Hungry Heart*. New American Library, New York.

Seidel, J.V. (1985) *The Ethnograph 2.0* (computer program). Qualis Research Associates, Littleton, Colorado.

Strauss, A. (1969) *Mirrors and Masks: The Search for Identity*. Sociology Press, California.

Stunkard, A.J. & Mahoney, M.J. (1976) Behavioral treatment of the eating disorders. In *Handbook of Behavior Modification and Behavior Therapy* (ed. H. Leitenberg). Appleton–Century–Crofts, New York.

VanItallie, T.B. (1979) Obesity: adverse effects on health and longevity. *American Journal of Clinical Nutrition*, **32**, 2723–33.

Weiss, A.R. (1977) Characteristics of successful weight reducers: a brief review of predictor variables. *Addictive Behaviors*, **2**, 193–201.

White, J.H. (1984) The process of embarking on a weight control program. *Health Care for Women International*, **5**, 77–91.

Wilson, G.T., & Brownwell, K.D. (1980) Behavior therapy for obesity: an evaluation of treatment outcome. *Behavior Research and Therapy*, **3**, 49–86.

Wineman, N. (1980) Obesity: locus of control, body image, weight loss and age at onset. *Nursing Research*, **29**, 231–7.

Wooley, S. & Wooley, O. (1984) Should obesity be treated at all? In *Eating and its Disorders* (eds. A. Stunkard & E. Stellar). pp. 185–92. Raven, New York.

Chapter 4
Benevolence, a central moral concept derived from a grounded theory study of nursing decision making in psychiatric settings

KIM LÜTZÉN, *Dr Med.Sc.*

Lecturer, Stockholm School of Health and Caring Sciences, Department of Nursing, and Doctoral Candidate, Department of Psychiatry, Karolinska Institute

and CONNY NORDIN, *MD*

Associate Professor, Department of Psychiatry, Karolinska Institute, Huddinge University Hospital, Huddinge, Sweden

Fourteen experienced nurses participated in an explorative study aimed at describing the experiential aspects of moral decision making in psychiatric nursing practice. In-depth interviews were conducted according to the grounded theory method. These were transcribed, coded and categorized in order to generate conceptual categories. The concept of benevolence was identified as a central motivating factor in the nurses' own accounts of situations in which decisions were made on behalf of the patient. This seems to conceptualize the nurses' expressed aim to do that which is 'good' for the patient in responding to his or her vulnerability. This study indicates the need for further research into the subjective, experiential aspect of ethical decision making from a contextual perspective.

Introduction

The nurse in the psychiatric setting, by nature of her close proximity to the patient, is often faced with making decisions on behalf of the patient on an everyday basis. In a previous theory-generating study (Lützén, 1990), the concept 'moral sensing' was identified, which describes the nurse's moral sensitivity to actions which may threaten the psychiatric patient's integrity. This study also raised questions concerning experiential aspects; for example, the need to examine the role of intuition and feelings in ethical decision making.

However, earlier studies focusing on ethics in nursing practice have predominantly investigated the cognitive moral development of nurses (for example, Ketefian, 1988). Considering that psychiatric patients are in a vulnerable position, since their capacity for self-choice and self-determination is often impaired by mental illness (Kopelman, 1989), there are few studies focusing on the experiential aspect of ethical decision making in psychiatry.

A call for new research approaches to examine moral decision making in nursing has arisen mainly out of the 'ethics of care' perspective, introduced by Gilligan (Gilligan, 1982; Gilligan & Attanucci, 1988) and Noddings (1984). Nurse theorists have similarly emphasized the activity of caring as a moral dimension and pointed out the need for developing conceptual models congruent to the lived experience of nursing practice (Benner, 1991; Watson, 1990).

Viewing the concept of 'care' in a phenomenological ethical framework points to the need to examine how moral competency is related to 'caring'. Shogan (1988), from a psychological perspective, examines the relationship of care to moral motivation and by doing so places an emphasis on character traits, emotion and relationships.

Fundamental to phenomenological ethics (Bengtsson, 1989; Tymeniecka, 1986; 1987, Lögstrup, 1971) is understanding the subjective experience rather than focusing only on objective and abstract reasoning. Similarly, the recently explicated ethics of care are relational and concrete, not impersonal and abstract. 'Caring' presupposes engagement and thus its area of investigation is choices within the relational context (Noddings, 1984; Cooper, 1990).

The study

The purpose of this present study is to investigate the experience of moral decision making in psychiatric nursing practice. The initial research question posed was: how does the nurse in the psychiatric setting experience making decisions for the patient on an everyday basis?

During the process of data analysis, more specific questions pertaining to the nurses' individual experiences were raised; for example, what factors influence the decisions made and how does each nurse motivate these decisions?

Method

Sample

Participants were selected based on two main criteria: more than five years' experience in psychiatry and willingness to share their experiences. The nurses who participated were suggested by nurses known to one of the authors (K.L.) and were described as 'competent' and 'reflective' in their work.

Fourteen nurses, 11 women and three men, were included. All had advanced education in psychiatric nursing. Ten were employed in hospital settings and four in community clinics at the time of the interviews. The study was approved by ethics committees in Gothenburg and Stockholm.

Data collection

Data were obtained from the transcriptions of face-to-face interviews, lasting from one to two hours. The focus of the interview was to discover commonalities in the way of responding to perceived patients' needs rather than to identify specific conflicts. The grounded theory approach (Glaser & Strauss, 1967; Strauss & Corbin, 1990) allowed for flexibility in the interview situation in that additional and clarifying questions could be posed.

The interviews began by allowing each nurse to describe an experience of making a decision concerning patient care where she/he had difficulty knowing what was right.

Data analysis

Analysis of data commenced with the first interview, searching for codes and some initial categories (Chenitz & Swanson, 1986). The Ethnograph, a computerized program for qualitative analysis, was used only in the first and second level of analysis allowing for comparison of codes and categories. In the third level of analysis, categories were integrated and their relationships defined.

Glaser's (1978) 'dimension family' was adopted in order to give structure to the analysis. In the dimension family, the notion of a whole is divided into parts with each part overlapping rather than being mutually exclusive. The goal is to identify a core category. In some studies, more than one category can be abstracted. According to Strauss & Corbin (1990), the analyst attempts to structure the theory with one central concept in relation to other concepts which are subsidiary. This strategy was adopted in the study.

Findings

The findings in this study generated the core category, structuring moral meaning, which describes the nurses' ways of interpreting a conflict within the nurse–patient framework and the subsidiary category, expressing benevolence. This chapter is limited to discussing the concept expressing benevolence and its dimensions, sensing the patient's vulnerability, responding to the patient's vulnerability and taking risks. 'Structuring moral meaning' is not discussed.

Expressing benevolence

Benevolence, in this study, is defined as the wish to do good compared to beneficence which is the practice of doing good (Seedhouse, 1988). The meaning of 'good' here is used to describe the intention underlying the nurse's actions, initiated by the nurse but affecting the patient in a concrete situation. The intention to do what is best in terms of the patient's well-being was explicitly as well as implicitly voiced by the nurses in their recapitulations of significant events.

Benevolence appeared as the nurses' genuine intentions, verbally expressed, to do that which is judged to be 'good' for the 'other'; in this context, the psychiatric patient. This genuine motivation can be exemplified by one of the nurses who worked on a psychogeriatric ward.

'I have always loved older people, how they think and are as individuals, not only as psychiatric patients.'

The same nurse continues:

'Being really close to a patient, to share his sorrow and problems, is a great privilege I have as a psychiatric nurse.'

The expressions 'have always loved older people' and 'being close' indicate that this nurse is capable as well as motivated to 'love' in the moral sense of the word. 'Being close to' and 'sharing' appear to express the nurse's motivation to care for the patient, based more on compassion and less on following the rule of obligation.

Two imperatives

The nurses in this study seem to face the challenge of dealing with two imperatives. One is interpreting the moral demand as expressed by the patient. The other is to act according to medical knowledge, as formalized by the physician. If both these imperatives coincide, then in essence there would be no conflict. But it seemed that the nurses who participated in this study felt a type of impulse arising from a moral conscience, creating an inner conflict between professional responsibility to follow rules and the personal moral commitment to care about the patient.

The explicit and implicit use of words such as 'comfort', 'feel for' and 'love' indicates that the nurses care 'about' the patient. Yet, caring 'about' the patient seemed to be integrated with many caring 'for' activities, for example, giving medication, bathing and feeding the patient.

For the nurses in this study, the expression of benevolence seemed to be linked to values and beliefs underpinning nursing ideology. In keeping with ideals of nursing, caring was made explicit by the nurses' awareness of the patient's integrity and factors which may influence his or her well-being. As one nurse described:

'When you work with older people, you have to deal with the reality of their dying and need for comfort and a home-like environment. It is so important that my patients feel a comforting hand from someone they trust and know. My role as a psychiatric nurse is to do something good for the patient's life, make the best of the situation; I can't let them down.'

Sensing the patient's vulnerability

Being vulnerable is defined here as being exposed and unprotected. It implies an unequal position between the nurse and the patient. 'Sensing' is used here to mean understanding and being aware of the patient's vulnerability without receiving any direct information.

Sensing the patient's vulnerability implies that the nurse has evaluated the situation and interpreted the moral meaning from the perspective of the patient's individual needs. Sensing the patient's vulnerable position appears to be based on an understanding of how the context can threaten a patient's integrity. An example follows:

'An incidence I remember well is about a patient, a very depressed patient. Our ward followed the principle which focused on building up the patient's own responsibility. Well, this patient hated himself, was very inactive. The main problem was that he refused to wash himself. My conflict was, should I force him to wash? He smelled and I knew that he would never allow this to happen if he were well. I wanted to protect his integrity, which would be threatened no matter what I did.'

Another situation where the nurse 'sensed the patient's vulnerability' concerned a young, female patient who could not communicate her situation because of language difficulties. This nurse believed that the patient's behaviour was misinterpreted by the physician who diagnosed the patient's behaviour as a 'psychotic reaction'. The nurse, according to her own account, attempted to see the whole situation this woman faced and thereby developed a contextual understanding. The nurse interpreted the patient as being in a crisis reinforced by communication problems and subsequent social isolation:

'I felt that the patient was misunderstood. She had no one except her husband, and he wanted her committed. I wanted to protect her. This I felt stronger than the physician's orders to give her an injection against her will. I saw myself on the side of the patient; she had no one to speak for her.'

The problem of trying to understand the vulnerable patient's needs and wishes is also illustrated in the account of a nurse who experienced a conflict when she reluctantly forced an older, confused female patient to shower:

'It did not feel right. The patient had no way of communicating to us what she feared. She couldn't decide herself if she wanted to wash; we did that for her.'

Applying the term 'sensing' in this study points to the way intuition and feelings dominated the nurses' interpretations of each situation. It appeared as if the nurses could, in a way, experience feelings that were different from their own.

Responding to the patient's vulnerability

The dimension 'responding to the patient's vulnerability' was indicated by the nurses' descriptions of how they interpreted and responded to the patients' needs. The difficulty, experienced in some situations, was not getting a positive response from the patient. An example is the nurse who described her experience with severely psychotic patients who fought even when she attempted to give comfort:

'Here on this ward you always get hit by the patients when you try to feed them, take them to the toilet. You can't help them with anything without getting clobbered. But they are so helpless, you can't just leave them. You have to use force in order for them to survive.'

The nurse in the above situation responded to the patient's vulnerability by choosing the alternative, 'to use force', because 'leaving them alone would be more unethical in the long run than forcing them, since they cannot take care of themselves'. As revealed in the above account, 'positive enjoyment' cannot always be the impulse for doing that which is good, at least not the immediate feeling.

Responding to the patient's vulnerability does not necessarily lead to similar actions. What seems to be similar is the nurses' sense of moral responsibility in accounting for the actions taken. In the situation where the nurse attempted to protect the patient who could not speak the language, her refusal to give the medication by force indicated a moral position. The nurse said:

'I wanted to protect her integrity as a person, and was prepared to take responsibility for my decision.'

Both the nurse who refused to go through with an action which she conceived as morally wrong (giving medication by force) and the nurse who felt she needed to use force in order to care for the patient's basic needs, took moral responsibility for their actions.

Upholding a trusting relationship was also identified as being part of responding to the vulnerability of the patient. For example, as one nurse explained:

'I try to be as honest as possible, thinking about the patient's situation and our relationship. The conflict for me was, should I get help or deal with the situation alone? I was afraid of making the wrong decision. I did not know whether getting help would cause him to lose faith in me. But, the important thing was to act, to respond to his needs. Not to act would be unethical for me.'

The nurse in this example attempted to see the patient's situation from his perspective before she could decide which response would be best in the specific situation. This shows that the main source of moral conflict as well as focus for attention seemed to be embedded in the interpersonal nurse–patient relationship, leading to the nurse's dilemma – how best to respond to the patient's vulnerability.

Taking risks

The dimension 'taking risks' refers to the tendency of the nurse to place her professional role in jeopardy if the wrong alternative is chosen. Two main types of risk taking are breaking rules, such as disputing the doctor's orders, and not following guidelines for practice. Both of these strategies could be linked to the nurse's motivation to do good when responding to the patient's vulnerable position.

An example of taking risks is illustrated by the following example of a nurse who did not follow the physician's orders to help him resuscitate an old, dying patient who had been a patient for a long time on the same psychiatric ward owing to a chronic illness. This nurse explains her actions:

'The patient was old. I had taken care of him on this ward for a long time. I knew his family. He had a right to end his days in peace.'

The nurse was conscious of not following the rules and that she could lose her job and her licence, but she felt a stronger unspoken demand to 'protect' the patient from unnecessary suffering. This nurse was respected by her staff and was described as being compassionate. She had worked on the ward for a long time and knew all of the patients well. The nurse was aware that she had overstepped her boundaries, in not co-operating with the physician. As it turned out, the situation was resolved but shows the dilemma between knowing that which is 'right' (judicially as well as ethically) and doing that which is 'good', a personal choice.

Discussion

In this study, normal decision making within the framework of the nurse–patient relationship seemed to be spurred by the 'benevolent sentiment', that is, the nurse's desire to do good within a concrete situation. The nurses' voiced intention to do 'good' was the main theme in all of the interviews. The benevolent sentiment may be a pertinent characteristic of moral comportment in psychiatric nursing care. A strong sense of benevolence could account for why some nurses choose to work in clinical areas where at times their efforts seem to be ungratifying.

Gilligan & Attanucci (1988) point out that the phenomenon of 'love' is tied to the activities of relationship and premised on the responsiveness of human connection. Similarly, the expression of 'love' in the form of attachment and attention are viewed by Murdoch (1970) as moral acts.

Similarly, Beauchamp & Childress (1989) suggest that a person who acts out of a sense of compassion is more likely to have 'morally good intentions' and be one we tend to trust. A person who only follows the rule of obligation could be satisfying external standards of conduct without a genuine regard for the patient's vulnerability.

Duty and morally good

From this perspective, a distinction can be made between the duty to follow that which is defined as medically right, as objectively interpreted by the physician, and that which is morally good, according to interpretations of what the patient would want (Beauchamp & Childress 1989).

Shogan (1988) points out that those in the 'helping professions' care for others as part of their work responsibilities. However, in defining motivation to 'care', Shogan makes a distinction between caring for, as a practical and technical activity, and caring about another's welfare. If a nurse cares about the patient's welfare she is likely to be genuinely motivated to do that which she perceives as being 'good'.

'Benevolence' is often viewed as a virtue, when a person conforms to a high standard of moral character or a praised moral ideal such as justice, wisdom, etc. (see McIntyre, 1985). However, the term 'virtue' is closely related to the term 'excellence', used in the nursing literature to denote a high standard of personal competency and knowledge (Benner, 1984). Charity, compassion and empathy, linked to benevolence, are character traits or qualities associated with virtue (Beauchamp & Childress, 1989), traits which are also seen in this study.

However, as McIntyre (1985) points out, definitions of what is considered a virtue change depending on the social as well as the historical context. Congruently, expressing benevolence in one (nursing) context can mean, for example, the conscientious adherence to rules and principles and, in another context, taking risks or transcending the rules and principles.

One could assume that a patient's integrity and well-being is not only dependent on right actions but also on the nurse's *desire* to do good. A question that may be raised for further research is, how does the patient respond or know if the nurse genuinely cares *about* him as an individual? It could be that a nurse who is trusted by the patient is one who not only acts based on principles of 'justice', but is also motivated to care by commitment, self-knowledge, empathy, compassion and responsibility.

Conflict

Sensing the vulnerable position of a patient may not always lead to satisfactory solutions of a moral conflict. Scudder & Bishop (1986) point out that two intentions of health care may come into conflict, namely the intention to carry out professional procedures and the intention to respond to the specific requests of a particular ill person. The nurse who believes she responds to the patient's unspoken request also has to deal with the organization's demand that medical procedures be followed. Thus taking risks in order to 'protect' the patient may lead to serious consequences for the patient as well as the nurse. Overstepping professional competency, such as misjudging the seriousness of a suicide threat, may result in the patient dying and the nurse losing her licence.

Scudder & Bishop (1986) maintain that benevolent actions which are morally good are 'accompanied by enjoyment – good actions produce positive enjoyment and evil actions, negative feelings'.

Responding to the patient's vulnerability can be compared with Gilligan's 'morality of response and care' (Gilligan & Attanucci, 1988). This means that 'moral problems are generally construed as issues of relationships or response. How to respond to others is resolved through the activity of care'.

Whether the expression of benevolence, derived in this study, is an essential motivational factor in moral decision making in psychiatric nursing needs to be examined further. The nurses in this study were specifically asked to relate one situation. Chinn (1991) suggests that a caring act carried out by one person to benefit another both influences and is influenced by the social context in which the act occurs. Can we then assume that genuine care derived from one described experience is not an isolated situation but reflects a personal characteristic constant over time and present in all types of situations?

Conclusion

According to the aim of the study, the expressed feelings may not reflect 'true' experiences in the sense that time, reflection and norms may have served as filters.

However, the nurses' own accounts of their actions in each situation must be seen as indications of moral motivation. The findings in this study also support the relevance of contextual approach to ethics.

As Hoffmaster (1990) points out, a 'contextualist morality' strives for a 'nuanced understanding of the practice of morality'. This means that a framework of rules and principle serving to justify actions from rational argument must be viewed in relationship to the type of concerns the nurses in this study have experienced.

References

Beauchamp, T.L. & Childress, J.F. (1989) *Principles of Biomedical Ethics*. Oxford University Press, Oxford.

Bengtsson, J. (1989) Det Högsta praktiska goda och det etiska kravet (The highest practical good and the ethical demand). In *Cum Grano Sales*, Gothenburg. Acta Philosophica Gothenburgensia.

Benner, P. (1984) *From Novice to Expert*. Addison-Wesley, Menlo Park, California.

Benner, P. (1991) The role of experience, narrative, and community in skilled ethical comportment. *Advances in Nursing Sciences*, **14**(2), 1–21.

Chenitz, C. & Swanson, J.M. (1986) *From Practice to Grounded Theory*. Addison-Wesley, Menlo Park, California.

Chinn, P. (1991) *Anthology on Caring*. National League for Nursing Press, New York.

Cooper, M.C. (1990) Reconceptualizing nursing ethics. *Scholarly Inquiry for Nursing Practice: An International Journal*, **4**(3), 209–18.

Gilligan, C. (1982) *In a Different Voice*. Harvard University Press, Cambridge, Massachusetts.

Gilligan, C. & Attanucci, J. (1988) Two moral orientations. In *Mapping the Moral Domain* (eds. C. Gilligan, J. Ward & J. McLean Taylor). Harvard University Press, Cambridge, Massachusetts.

Glaser, B. (1978) *Theoretical Sensitivity*. The Sociology Press, Mill Valley, California.

Glaser, B. & Strauss, A. (1967) *The Discovery of Grounded Theory*. Aldine de Gruyter, New York.

Hoffmaster, B. (1990) Morality and the Social Sciences. In *Social Science Perspectives on Medical Ethics* (ed. G. Weiz), pp. 241–60. Kluwer Academic, Boston.

Ketefian, S. (1988) *Moral Reasoning and Ethical Practice in Nursing: An Integrative Review*. National League for Nursing Press, New York.

Kopelman, L. (1989) Moral problems in psychiatry. In *Medical Ethics* (ed. R. Veatch) pp. 254–89. Jones and Bartlett, Boston.

Lögstrup, K. (1971) *The Ethical Demand*. Fortress Press, Philadelphia.

Lützén, K. (1990) Moral sensing and ideological conflict: aspects of the therapeutic relationship in psychiatric nursing. *Scandinavian Journal of Caring Sciences*, **4**(2), 69–76.

McIntyre, A. (1985) *After Virtue*. Duckworth, London.

Murdoch, I. (1970) *The Sovereignty of God*. Cox & Wyman, London.

Noddings, N. (1984) *Caring, A Feminine Approach to Ethics*. USCF Press, Berkeley, California.

Scudder, J. & Bishop, A. (1986) The moral sense and health care. In *Analecta Husserliana* (ed. A.T. Tymeniecka), **20**, 125–58. Reidel, Dordrecht, The Netherlands.

Seedhouse, D. (1988) *Ethics, The Heart of Health Care*. John Wiley and Sons, Chichester.

Shogan, D. (1988) *Care and Moral Motivation*. OISE Press, Toronto.

Strauss, A. & Corbin, J. (1990) *Basics of Qualitative Research*. Sage, Newbury Park, California.

Tymeniecka, A. (1986) The moral sense and the human person within the fabric of communal life. In *Analecta Husserliana*, **20**, 3–44. Reidel, Dordrecht, The Netherlands.

Tymeniecka, A. (1987) Morality and the life-world or the moral sense within the world of life. In *Analecta Husserliana*, **22**, 3–13. Reidel, Dordrecht, The Netherlands.

Watson, J. (1990) The moral failure of the patriarchy. *Nursing Outlook*, **38**(2), 62–7.

Chapter 5
Mid-range theory building and the nursing theory–practice gap: a respite care case study

MIKE NOLAN, *BEd, MA, MSc, PhD, RMN, RGN*
Senior Lecturer in Nursing Research, Health Studies Research Division

and GORDON GRANT, *BSc, MSc, PhD*
Director, Centre for Social Policy Research and Development, University of Wales, Bangor, Gwynedd, Wales

Nursing, with its historical roots in practice, has tended to have an uneasy relationship with theory. Whilst the benefits of theory to nursing have been propounded by many commentators, it remains that theory all too rarely informs nursing practice. This chapter argues for the development and utilization of mid-range theories as representing a solution to this problem. The advantages of such an approach are illustrated by the application, testing and refinement of Chenitz's theory of relocation to a hospital-based respite care scheme for the frail elderly.

Introduction

At first sight it appears to be a relatively easy matter to present a case for the positive contribution theory has made to the development of nursing. The literature offers seductive arguments extolling the virtues of theory and its potential for building a unique body of knowledge to enhance the professional status of nursing, facilitate communication between practitioners and improve patient care (McFarlane, 1976; Craig, 1980; Walker & Avant, 1983; Torres, 1990; Meleis, 1991; Chinn & Krammer 1991). Kenny (1992) provides a detailed list of these putative benefits.

It is in particular the contribution of theory to the improvement of patient care which is held to be the ultimate benefit of theory to a practice discipline such as nursing since, by the practical application of theories, nursing action might be rendered more efficient and effective (Chinn & Krammer, 1991; Meleis, 1991; Ingram 1991).

Recently, writers (Moore, 1990; Girot, 1990; Draper, 1990; Ingram, 1991, Kenny 1992, Robinson 1992) have reflected upon and questioned the role and value of nursing theory to the development of nursing in general and nursing practice in particular. Such evidence suggests that theory cannot be said to have facilitated communication given the 'utter semantic confusion' (McFarlane, 1976) created by the conflicting use of terms, a situation which hardly seems to have improved with conceptual distinctions remaining 'hair-splitting, unclear and confusing' (Meleis, 1991).

If theorists themselves find such aspects difficult to unravel, practitioners have often reacted by rejecting theory itself. This has resulted in what has been termed the theory–practice gap (Craig, 1980; Miller, 1985; Gruending, 1985; Clarke, 1986), with the rift now being so wide that it has been referred to as a 'chasm' (Lewis, 1988). Resultant debates have tended to develop into a vicious circle, with theorists berating practitioners for their lack of concern with the conceptual basis for their actions, whilst practitioners bemoan theoretical approaches which are seen as having little or no relevance to their daily work.

Theory related to practice

Miller (1985) argues that if it is virtually impossible for experienced nurses to relate theory to their practice then there is something wrong with either theory or practice. Draper (1990) has no such doubts and lays the blame fairly and squarely with theory. The root of, and possible solution to, this problem appears to lie in the scope and abstraction of many nursing theories.

Kitson (1985) contends that in attempting to develop a unified theory which offers both professional status and scientific credibility, nursing has tended to overstate itself with theories which, at a stroke, purport to offer the answers to all life's questions. As a consequence, such theories have been too complex, global, abstract and esoteric for practitioners and are seen as having nothing to offer to their immediate areas of concern (Miller, 1985; Meleis & Price, 1988; Schmieding, 1990; Girot, 1990; Chinn & Krammer, 1991; Ingram, 1991, Reed & Robbins, 1991; Kenny, 1992). Whilst the impracticality of unified approaches has been noted for some time (McFarlane, 1976), it is still considered that many theories, in their efforts to explain everything, succeed only in explaining nothing (Draper, 1990). Therefore, as Kenny (1992) points out, the use of theories and models in nursing has resulted in sweeping generalizations which 'are not always personally, culturally or contextually appropriate'.

In overcoming this difficulty many authors advocate that theories of lesser scope and abstraction are considered (McFarlane, 1976; Clarke, 1986; Draper, 1990; Moore, 1990; Ingram, 1991; Reid & Bond, 1991). Such theories have been termed 'mid-range' and address a more limited number of variables in particular situations (scope), whilst being empirically grounded and focusing on practical problems (abstraction) (Rogers & Shoemaker,

1971; Walker & Avant, 1983; Fawcett, 1984; Lowenberg, 1984). According to Clarke (1986), mid-range theories should appeal to practitioners as being more directly accessible conceptually and linguistically. Reed & Robbins (1991) contend that, given the diversity of nursing practice, the search for grand theory is inappropriate and nursing would be better served by developing mid-range theories that are 'more precisely stated, more easily treated and produce more specific indications for practice'.

A recent research study afforded the authors the opportunity to apply and test just such a theory in a particular situation and to reflect upon the value of mid-range theories in narrowing the theory–practice gap. The situation in question was the use of hospital accommodation to provide respite care for carers of the frail elderly.

Applying a mid-range theory

Recent British community care policies have highlighted the need for statutory services to support informal carers and have advocated that domiciliary, day and respite care services should be developed in order to achieve this aim (Department of Health, 1989). Despite the assumption that respite care is a 'good thing' a recent literature review (Nolan, 1991) suggested that previous conceptualizations of the benefits of respite care have been limited, focusing mainly on instrumental outcomes for carers themselves.

Therefore, the main purpose of respite care is described largely in terms of maintaining carers in their role and the provision of the break is seen as sufficient to achieve this end. Relatively little attention has been given to the wider potential of respite care for addressing carers' other needs, for example for information, skills training and emotional support. Even less attention appears to have been devoted to the impact of such services on elderly dependants admitted for the break.

Nevertheless, the literature indicates that many carers experience profound feelings of guilt at using respite services and that the reaction of the dependant to the admission is one of the key variables mediating such guilt. It follows that if respite care can be made a positive experience for the user than carer guilt is potentially lessened and the benefits for both parties heightened.

In a study seeking to explicate the benefits of a hospital-based rota bed system in a defined geographical location, it was reasoned that nurses, as the prime providers of care, should consider ways in which to understand the impact of respite care on the elderly users. Therefore, one of the aims of the study was to identify those factors which might differentiate between a positive and a negative reaction by the dependants to the service.

Chenitz's theory

Institutional respite care, especially that based on a rota, involves the regular and repeated movement of the elderly user between home and hospital. The literature addresses such an issue under the general title of 'relocation effects'. A search of the relocation literature identified a theory which seemed to offer an explanation of such relocation effects.

The theory in question is that of Chenitz (1983). Chenitz, in developing this theory, intended that it should guide nursing action by fulfilling two basic prerequisites: that it should frame information with enough specificity to guide practice in particular situations, whilst being generalizable to a variety of similar situations with differing individuals. It is the application of this theory to a respite care situation and a test of its generalizability which forms the main part of this chapter.

Relocation effects: a theoretical explanation

Using a grounded theory methodology and a combination of observations, interviews and documentary analysis, Chenitz (1983) studied the process of adjustment of 30 older people following admission to two nursing homes. Data were collected longitudinally from the time of admission until six to nine months later. Based on her analysis, Chenitz (1983) argues that underlying individual reactions to relocation are certain common elements or basic conditions, the unique combination of which determines people's subsequent behaviour and whether they accept or resist the admission.

The first of these basic conditions is contextualizing variables surrounding the event. These include both generally held beliefs about the families' responsibility to care and also the specific nature of the particular family relationships. These frame the event and set the stage.

Basic conditions

Other basic conditions identified in the theory are as follows:

(1) Centrality or the importance of the event in terms of the older individual's struggle to retain independence and an element of control in their lives.
(2) Desirability or the extent to which the move is seen as being desirable and to the personal advantage of the individual in contrast to being associated with being unwanted and dependent.
(3) Legitimation or whether there is a plausible and legitimate reason for the move.
(4) Participation in decision making and the extent to which the admission is

seen as being voluntary. Chenitz (1983) argues that if desirability can be married with legitimation then it is possible for the older person to construct a perception of the admission as being a personal choice, even if in reality it is not.

(5) Temporality, i.e. the timing of the admission, one of the key concepts here being the extent to which it is seen as being reversible.

The theory suggests that adverse relocation effects are most pronounced where the admission combines irreversibility with undesirability, a lack of personal choice and no legitimating circumstances. However, it is also argued that negative effects can be ameliorated when some of the basic conditions are met.

In describing the possible reactions to admission, Chenitz (1983) uses two broad categories which are further divided into two subcategories. Thus people may either accept or resist the move into care.

Acceptance is achieved either by strategic submission or submission by default. The former usually occurs when the admission is reversible and therefore accepted for a time-limited period, or alternatively when the individual is able to perceive the event as a considered choice from amongst a very restricted range of options. Submission by default normally follows a catastrophic life event, for example the death of a spouse, when the admission is not seen as the most significant factor.

Resistance is likely to occur when one or more of the basic conditions are not met and may be either resigned-resisting or forceful-resisting. The former is characterized by withdrawal and apathy, a reaction which results in guilt and anger amongst any family. The latter is, as the name suggests, a more active response involving deliberate failure to participate in the life of the home and possibly culminating in verbal and/or physical abuse.

Therefore, whilst very few people would probably make a deliberate choice to go into respite care, Chenitz's (1983) theory does suggest ways in which the experience can be made more positive and potentially more beneficial. Respite care is not permanent and therefore meets the important basic condition of reversibility, a fact which should reduce anxiety to some extent. However, if it is to be of optimum benefit it is still necessary to provide a desirable and legitimate reason and to make the environment as positive as possible. In this area, respite care in hospitals can have a distinct advantage over other institutionally based services.

Many elderly people entering respite care in hospital often perceive themselves as being admitted for assessment and/or therapy and this may provide both a desirable and legitimate reason for admission. Therefore, while true choice may be absent it may still be possible for the person to perceive that the respite care admission is the result of a personal decision. Such a self-constructed perception of legitimation has been noted in relation to other similar services, for example day hospital care (Nolan, 1986).

In order to test the utility of Chenitz's (1983) theory in a respite care situation and to consider the extent to which it might help explain reactions to such care, semi-structured interviews were held with 30 elderly users in four locations. From a detailed content analysis of their responses it was apparent that Chenitz's theory, originally developed to account for reactions to admission to a nursing home, required further refinement and development in order that it might account for reactions to the qualitatively different form of admission that respite care afforded.

Perceptions of respite care

On the basis of the analysis, the perceptions of the elderly users of the respite beds can be neatly divided into three groups: beneficiaries, tolerators and abandoned.

Beneficiaries

The first group of users constituted about a quarter of those interviewed (7/30). They will be termed the beneficiaries, a particularly apt descriptor as for these individuals the respite admission was a most positive experience. The overall impression was that coming in had some perceived meaning and benefit for themselves. Whilst they saw the importance of the break for their carer, this was a secondary consideration as the main reason for the admission was described in terms of personal benefit. As such, the two weeks in every eight which they spent in hospital became an important and enjoyable part of their lives.

Typically, the admission afforded a perceived opportunity for treatment or at least reassessment. Moreover, most people in this group had been coming in for respite care for a number of years and had developed significant relationships with both staff and other respite users, thus ensuring an active and enjoyable respite stay.

On the basis of the above, the beneficiaries considered respite care to be a positive personal choice that was not only legitimate but also highly desirable. Moreover, these individuals had maintained excellent relationships with their carer(s) and therefore the contextualizing factors surrounding each admission were also positive. Thus, in terms of Chenitz's (1983) theory, all the basic conditions had been met and one would predict an acceptance of the admission.

However, whilst Chenitz's (1983) theory proved most useful in explaining the reactions of the beneficiaries, one of the basic conditions, temporality, requires some modification when the theory is applied to respite care. In Chenitz's (1983) original conceptualization, temporality referred mainly to the degree to which the admission was reversible. In relation to respite care, this is clearly the case. However, when applied to rota beds another consideration arises in that reversibility is combined with both predictability and regularity, in that both the duration of the admission and the timing of subsequent readmissions are known.

This adds another dimension, which the authors term anticipation. This was influential in determining the reactions of all the users of the respite care. Therefore, for the beneficiaries the rota bed stay was anticipated with pleasure and a positive reinforcement cycle was created. This helped to ensure that the next admission was anticipated with pleasure and therefore maintained the positive contextualizing factors surrounding the event.

It was also apparent from observations of staff contact with such individuals that they might be considered as 'favourites' whom staff would deliberately seek out to engage in conversation. It was not difficult to see why, as the researcher (M.N.) also enjoyed the interviews with these respondents who were socially adept and had interesting tales to tell. The positive staff contact further reinforced the favourable reaction of the beneficiaries.

As a consequence of the above, acceptance by the beneficiaries went beyond that suggested in Chenitz's (1983) original conceptualization. Therefore, acceptance was not by a process of mere submission, either strategically or by default, but involved a much more enthusiastic response. To describe this, the authors suggest the term embracing as better conveying the most positive acceptance of respite care by this particular group of users.

Tolerators

In contrast to the above group the largest number of users (17/30) are best described as tolerating the admission on the basis that it was for a time-limited period. The basic condition of temporality had been satisfied. However, as will be described below, the manner in which this group anticipated the admission differed considerably from the beneficiaries. Moreover, they also varied in other basic conditions.

Therefore, whilst they had maintained good relationships with their carers, they saw no benefit to themselves in accepting respite care. Rather they perceived that the respite admission was for the sole benefit of their carers. This provided a legitimate reason for respite care, but in contrast to the beneficiaries there was little evidence of desirability. This apart, they were not a homogeneous group, however, and can be further divided into three subgroups for which the authors have coined the terms, the endurers, the disillusioned and the martyrs.

Endurers

The largest subgroup (10/17) were the endurers. Such individuals put up with the respite admission for the benefit of their carers. They appreciated that the person looking after them both needed and deserved a break and, as outlined above, this provided a legitimate reason for them to accept the admission. Therefore, whilst not embracing the admission, acceptance and anticipation of respite care was by and large good humoured with no real resentment. It was appreciated that two weeks in hospital in every eight was a prime factor in maintaining them at home for the other six. A strong element of centrality was in evidence. However, there was little evidence of a positive effect on the self-esteem of this group.

Some found comfort in that sharing an environment with the long-stay patients made them realize that their own circumstances could be a lot worse. For others, however, this had the opposite effect and they found rather depressing the prospect that they themselves might end up in such an institution on a permanent basis.

A number of others made fairly mundane comments about the food being 'good' and the staff very 'nice', but most described long periods of boredom and inertia, with time hanging heavy on their hands. However, none felt that they could be critical as they were conscious that they would be returning again in six weeks. Moreover, whilst being sociable with both staff and patients, no really significant relationships had been forged with either group.

Therefore, whilst sufficient basic conditions were met for this subgroup to accept the admission, both positive choice and desirability were absent. However, they endured the admission and generally made the most of a bad job.

Disillusioned

A smaller subgroup (3/17) were the disillusioned. For these three people the respite care had been sold to them on the basis that it would afford an opportunity for further treatment. Whilst they still appreciated that the admission would provide a break for their carer, thus providing an element of legitimation, the prospect of benefit to themselves added desirability and also increased their sense of self-worth and hope. Thus, initially there was an element of positive anticipation. However, the hoped-for treatment did not materialize for these individuals and therefore the desirability was removed and there tended to be a reduction in self-esteem. This led to disillusionment. However, their good relationship with carers sustained an element of legitimation, and the centrality of the admission in terms of keeping the carer going was quite apparent.

For both the above groups the admission did not appear to have affected the quality of their relationship with their carers and there was a realization that their carer both needed and deserved a break. The time-limited nature of the admission made it tolerable, even though anticipation was on the whole negative.

'Well, let's say I put up with it. I know my wife needs the break and it's only for a fortnight. Mind you, if I thought I was here on a permanent basis I'd say "Give me the gun".'

In terms of acceptance, these groups therefore adopted what Chenitz (1983) termed a 'strategic submitting' stance.

Martyrs

There was also a third subgroup (4/17) who might be described as tolerating the admission. The overriding rationale for accepting respite care for such individuals was the realization that their carer needed a break. However, in contrast to the previous two subgroups there was an evident element of resentment amongst these individuals and they did not describe the break as being deserved.

Therefore, whilst those in this subgroup tolerated respite care because they felt refusal might lead to a collapse of the caring situation, they also felt as if their acceptance was a sacrifice made by them for the carer. They felt like martyrs. For the martyrs respite care seemed to threaten the more fragile relationship with their carer and anticipation tended to be in terms of a negative reinforcement cycle. The martyrs therefore were in danger of joining the third main group.

Abandoned

For the third group of users, the abandoned (6/30), the respite care was a totally negative experience with none of the basic conditions being met and it often resulted in a reduction in their perceived self-esteem. Such individuals saw no legitimate reason for the admission at all. They were aware that they were attending in order for their carer to have a break but did not consider that such a break was either needed or deserved. They therefore felt that they had been abandoned by their carers. They clearly saw that they had no choice in the decision to come in for care and deeply resented the fact that they perceived themselves as having been forced to accept it:

'I'm coming because they [doctor and staff] tell me that my daughter needs a break and if she can't get one then I'll have to go into a home. I've got no choice in the matter. It's like everything else, I always have to jump when she says so.'

These were most often the individuals who were described as manipulative, domineering and unappreciative by their carers. Therefore, for this group the respite admission served only to reinforce their poor relationship with their carer and anticipation of each admission created a negative reinforcement cycle resulting in a downward spiral.

The abandoned were much more likely to resist the admission, either by resigned resistance, that is largely passive withdrawal or more forceful means, typically refusal to co-operate and participate in the ward. This understandably had the added effect of making these individuals less popular with both other patients and staff, further compounding their already negative perceptions.

Mid-range theory building and nursing practice

It was suggested in the introduction that, in their search for a unified theory of nursing, the work of many nursing theorists has alienated rather than enthused practitioners. Mid-range theory was offered as a possible solution to this problem. By the application of Chenitz's (1983) theory of relocation to a qualitatively different form of admission and its subsequent revision, it is considered that the utility of the mid-range theory has been demonstrated.

Traditionally therefore, a theory is judged by its ability to describe, explain and predict the phenomena of interest. Ultimately, however, it is usually considered that nursing theory must also prescribe or act as a guide to nursing practice (McFarlane, 1976; Craig, 1980; Clarke, 1986; Walker & Avant, 1983; Draper, 1990; Torres, 1990; Chinn & Krammer, 1991; Ingram, 1991; Meleis, 1991).

The authors would contend that Chenitz's (1983) theory has demonstrated its ability to describe and explain. It also has the potential to predict which combination of circumstances would lead to respite care being accepted (either embraced or strategically) or resisted and, moreover, to suggest which nursing actions might ameliorate these reactions. As Meleis (1991) advocates, it provides a basis for the fundamental components of nursing practice: assessment, diagnosis, intervention and evaluation.

Positive attribute

The theory was developed and refined from a user perspective and this is increasingly seen as representing a positive attribute of future nursing theories. Previous theories have been criticized for their narrow professional focus which has often lacked a user or consumer dimension:

'Nursing models are the perspectives of nurses, of certain nurses. The perspective of the consumer does not enter into them, except as interpreted by the nurse theorist.'

Janforum (1986)

Thus, whilst it is argued that practice-informing theory should be developed inductively from the actions of nurses themselves (Clarke, 1986; Draper, 1990), some writers advocate that theories must take adequate account of both nurses' and users' views (Meleis, 1991), or even that the users' view be given the major consideration (Morse *et al.*, 1990).

Conclusion

If nursing's claim to act as the patient's advocate and to offer holistic care is to have any credibility, it is contended that the profession will need to adopt a balanced approach to their development. This may well require a far broader definition of what constitutes 'theory' (Sandelowski 1993) and will certainly necessitate the cultivation of an open and critical mind. Hence, suggestions that theories borrowed from other disciplines do not advance the cause of nursing in moving towards a unique body of knowledge (Draper, 1990) are, like the search for a unified theory, symptoms of the profession's own insecurities and are likely to lead to approaches which are merely self-serving. However, nursing must resist the temptation to adapt theoretical approaches without a consideration of their empirical support (Reed & Robbins 1991). Whilst the promise of a model which will both define and verify nursing is not without a certain appeal (Reed & Robbins 1991), recognition also needs to be given to the fact that it is only of use if it 'helps us to understand and negotiate our way around the nursing and health care world' (Robinson 1992). Grand theory does not appear to meet these criteria.

Far better for both nursing and the people it serves that McFarlane's (1976) advice be heeded and that efforts are directed towards the development of an eclectic knowledge base that derives its uniqueness from its application and testing in a nursing context. It has been suggested that this will require the definition, specification and refinement of key concepts as they apply to certain areas of practice (Robinson 1992, Nolan & Grant 1993). Only in this way will the reciprocal relationship between models and practice be facilitated in order that nursing knowledge 'guide and direct clinical services' (Fawcett 1992).

As has been demonstrated in this chapter, the building, testing and refining of appropriate mid-range theories, irrespective of their origin, provide a source of knowledge which is relevant to the real world of practice and understandable to those who live and work in it.

References

Chenitz, W.C. (1983) Entry into a nursing home as status passage: a theory to guide nursing practice. *Geriatric Nursing*, March/April, 92–7.

Chinn, P.L. & Krammer, K.M. (1991) *Theory and Nursing: A Systematic Approach*, 3rd edn. Mosby Year Book, St Louis.

Clarke, M. (1986) Action and reflection: practice and theory in nursing. *Journal of Advanced Nursing*, **11**, 3–11.

Craig, S.L. (1980) Theory development and its relevance for nursing, *Journal of Advanced Nursing*, **5**, 349–55.

Department of Health (1989) *Caring for People: Community Care in the Next Decade and Beyond*. HMSO, London.

Draper, P. (1990) The development of theory in British nursing: current position and future prospects. *Journal of Advanced Nursing*, **15**, 12–15.

Fawcett, J. (1984) *Analysis and Evaluation of Conceptual Models of Nursing*. F.A. Davies, Philadelphia.

Fawcett, J. (1992) Conceptual models and nursing practice: the reciprocal relationship. *Journal of Advanced Nursing*, **17**(2), 224–8.

Girot, E. (1990) Discussing nursing theory. *Senior Nurse*, **10**(6), 16–19.

Gruending, D.C. (1985) Nursing theory: a vehicle for professionalization. *Journal of Advanced Nursing*, **10**, 553–8.

Ingram, R. (1991) Why does nursing need theory? *Journal of Advanced Nursing*, **16**, 350–53.

Janforum (1986) Identifying the place of theoretical frameworks in an evolving discipline. *Journal of Advanced Nursing*, **11**, 103–7.

Kenny, T. (1992) Nursing models fail in practice. *British Journal of Nursing*, **2**(2), 133–6.

Kitson, A. (1985) Educating for quality. *Senior Nurse*, **3**(4), 11–16.

Lewis, T. (1988) Leaping the chasm between theory and practice. *Journal of Advanced Nursing*, **13**, 345–51.

Lowenberg, F.M. (1984) Professional ideology, middle range theories and knowledge building for social work practice. *British Journal of Social Work*, **14**, 309–22.

McFarlane, J.K. (1976) The role of research and the development of nursing theory. *Journal of Advanced Nursing*, **1**, 443–51.

Meleis, A.I. (1991) *Theoretical Nursing: Developments and Progress*, 2nd edn. Lippincott, Philadelphia.

Meleis, A.I. & Price, M.J. (1988) Strategies and conditions for teaching theoretical nursing: an international perspective. *Journal of Advanced Nursing*, **13**, 592–604.

Miller, A. (1985) The relationship between nursing theory and nursing practice. *Journal of Advanced Nursing*, **10**, 417–24.

Moore, S. (1990) Thoughts on the discipline of nursing as we approach the year 2000. *Journal of Advanced Nursing*, **15**, 825–8.

Morse, J.M., Solberg, S.M., Neander, W.L., Bottorff, J.L. & Johnson, J.L. (1990) Concepts of caring and caring as a concept *Advances in Nursing Science*, **13**(1), 1–14.

Nolan, M.R. (1986) Day care in perspective: a comparative study of two day hospitals for the elderly. Unpublished MA thesis. University of Wales, Bangor.

Nolan, M.R. (1991) Timeshare beds: a pluralistic evaluation of rota beds in continuing care hospitals. Unpublished PhD thesis. University of Wales, Bangor.

Nolan, M.R. & Grant, G. (1993) Rust-out and therapeutic reciprocity: concepts to advance the nursing care of older people. *Journal of Advanced Nursing*, **18**, 1305–14.

Reed, J. & Robbins, I. (1991) Models of nursing: their relevance to the care of elderly people. *Journal of Advanced Nursing*, **16**, 1350–7.

Reid, J. & Bond, S. (1991) Nurses' assessment of elderly patients in hospital. *International Journal of Nursing Studies*, **1**, 55–64.

Robinson, J. (1992) The problems with paradigms in a caring profession. *Journal of Advanced Nursing*, **17**, 632–8.

Rogers, E.M. & Shoemaker, F.F. (1971) *Communication of Innovations: A Cross-cultural Approach*, 2nd edn. Free Press, New York.

Sandelowski, M. (1993) Theory unmasked: the uses of and guises of theory in qualitative research. *Research in Nursing and Health*, **16**, 213–18.

Schmieding, N.J. (1990) An integrative nursing theoretical framework. *Journal of Advanced Nursing*, **15**, 463–467.

Torres, G. (1990) The place of concepts and theories within nursing. In *Nursing Theories: The Base for Professional Nursing Practice*, 3rd edn (ed. J.B. George). Prentice Hall International, New Jersey.

Walker, L.O. & Avant, K.C. (1983) *Strategies for Theory Construction in Nursing*. Appleton–Century–Crofts, Norwalk, Connecticut.

Chapter 6
Toward a theory of touch: the touching process and acquiring a touching style

CAROLE A. ESTABROOKS, *MN, RN*
Doctoral Student, Faculty of Nursing, University of Alberta, Edmonton, Alberta, Canada

and JANICE M. MORSE, *PhD(Anthro), PhD (Nurs), RN*
Professor, School of Nursing, The Pennsylvania State University, University Park, Pennsylvania, USA

Methods of grounded theory were used to explore the questions: How do intensive care nurses perceive touch and the process of touching? How do intensive care nurses learn to touch? Data were collected by in-depth interviews with eight experienced intensive care nurses from the same intensive care unit of a large urban Canadian hospital. Findings revealed two substantive processes, the touching process and acquiring a touching style, neither of which has been previously reported. The stages and phases of these processes are described as well as cueing, the core variable. Based on the data analysis, touch was conceptualized as a gestalt with multiple dimensions, suggesting that valid operational definitions of touch must incorporate more than skin-to-skin contact.

Neglected area in nursing research

One of the most neglected areas in nursing research is the investigation of the touch behaviours of nurses, more specifically, the study of touching itself and how it is learned. This gap is extraordinary in a profession in which the touching of others is integral to the provision of nursing care. In this study, touch does not refer to therapeutic touch (Krieger, 1975), but rather to touch that occurs day-to-day in the course of normal nursing activities.

Nurses have the permission of society to violate norms, and touching others intimately is a component in the routine accomplishment of many nursing tasks. In the delivery of this care, nurses enter into a reciprocal equation, the nurse–patient relationship. In this relationship, touching is central. Our ability to provide care effectively, whether that care be for patient or nurse, is at least partially dependent on our understanding of the mechanisms of touch. In this chapter, findings relevant to the nurse in the touch interaction are addressed, including antecedents to the touching behaviours of nurses.

Few studies

Few studies exist that report findings specifically related to the touching behaviours of nurses. Those that do exist do not address how nurses learn to touch or, more fundamentally, how nurses touch, that is, the specific mechanisms of the touching process. Researchers who have previously investigated touching behaviours of nurses have largely used non-participant observational methods, most often attempting to correlate frequency of touch with various nurse and patient characteristics (Barnett, 1972; Clement, 1983; De Wever, 1977; El-Kafass, 1983; Mitchell *et al.*, 1985; Watson, 1975). The results of these studies have not been consistent, and statistically significant correlations are frequently not reported. These studies are subject to the inherent problems of accurately observing and recording touch, to problems of superficial analysis, and to the failure to use reliable instruments or instruments yielding results comparable across studies (Porter *et al.*, 1986). Moreover, a troubling question is raised, in that this research provides superficial information about 'who touches whom, where and how often ... [but] little is known about the meanings conveyed' (Jones & Yarbrough, 1985).

The 'touching style' of nurses was referred to by Weiss (1986) and implicit references to it can be drawn from the work of others. However, until this study touching style had not been studied to any degree. Recently, Bottorff (1992) made an important further contribution to the study of nurses' touching styles by identifying four types of *attending* which represent styles used by nurses during nurse–patient interactions involving touch. Touching style is the amount and kind of touch that a nurse uses in her practice. It is learned and, additionally, it is mediated by complex contextual factors.

Previous work on touch has generally identified two kinds of touch:

(1) Caring (Clement, 1987; Glick, 1986) or comforting touch (Morse, 1983; Weiss, 1986).
(2) Task (Burnside, 1981) or procedural touch (Clement, 1983; Glick, 1986; Mitchell *et al.*, 1985; Weiss, 1986).

This literature implies that the use of high amounts of caring touch is 'good'; that is, certain styles of touching are better than others. Using the methods of ethnoscience, Estabrooks (1989) identified a third kind of touch, that is, touch used to protect the nurse and/or the patient. This protective touch has controlling and distancing characteristics that frequently elicit negative feelings in both nurses and patients.

Estabrooks (1989) also reports normative patterns of touch among nurses in an intensive care unit (ICU), identifying the five types of nurses, each with a particular style of touching relating to the amount and kind of touch they used. She also describes findings that suggest one dimension of learning to touch is related to variables that are context-bound, such as patient characteristics, environmental conditions, and the beliefs and values of a particular subculture. These normative patterns explain situational variation in a nurse's touching style and offer insights into the complexity and number of factors that influence touching behaviour.

Two researchers have proposed theoretical frameworks, within which are implicit references to processes of touch. In 1979, Weiss proposed 'a continuum of tactile arousal', and in 1986 she introduced a model of 'factors influencing the effect of caregiver touch on the incidence of dysrhythmia'. Pepler (1984) proposed a framework of 'concepts related to touch as comforting', which suggests five sequential phases with feedback mechanisms: patient behaviour, nurse behaviour, nurse–patient interaction, patient response, and nurse response.

Poorly understood concept

One of the most salient problems in the study of touch is that the concept itself is poorly understood (Estabrooks, 1987). Observational studies that are conducted deductively define touch as an observable skin-to-skin contact. Yet, if touch is essential to have a communicative, affective dimension, then the limitation of observational methods is immediately apparent. Although some researchers have attempted to understand touch by interviewing the patient (Birch, 1986; Penny, 1979), these studies have been limited by retrospective interviews. A study in which nurses served as the primary informants could not be found.

Purpose of the study

The purpose of this study was to examine touch from the perspective of nurses employed in an intensive care setting. The first part of the study examined the structure of touch and touching norms in an ICU (Estabrooks, 1989). The second part of the study (reported in this chapter) examined the process of touching. Data collection for part two of the study was guided by the following questions:

(1) How do intensive care nurses learn to touch, that is, acquire a touching style?
(2) How do intensive care nurses perceive touch and the process of touching?

Methods

The ICU was conceptualized as a discreet cultural system with its own norms for behaviour. Grounded theory methods (Glaser & Strauss, 1967; Glaser, 1978) were used to analyse the data; these methods enabled the identification of two substantive processes: acquiring a touching style, and the basic social process of touching, as well as a core variable, cuing.

Sample

A purposive sample consisting of eight experienced ICU staff nurses was selected from the same general systems ICU of a large urban Canadian hospital. Informants ranged in age from 26 to 47 years and were all Caucasian and female. The number of years in ICU ranged from four to ten, with a mean of seven years. Four of the informants held a diploma in nursing, and four had a baccalaureate degree in nursing. All of the informants were self-described 'touchers' who believed that touch was important to people and to nursing. One informant withdrew from the study after the second interview due to a geographic move.

Data collection and analysis

Data were collected by in-depth interviews. Interactive interviews were conducted at least three times with each informant over a five-month period. Three of the informants participated in a group interview near the end of the data collection period.

In the first interview, which was unstructured, the meaning and use of touch was elicited through the use of broad questions. Informants were asked: 'Could you begin by talking about touch in the ICU?' 'Could you describe how touch is used by ICU nurses?' 'How do you use touch in caring for your patients?' 'Do different nurses touch differently?' The second and third interviews were more structured and consisted of filling in 'thin' areas of the data, elaborating on ideas and concepts, and exploring new areas. In the final group interview, concepts and models were verified with the informants. Data analysis proceeded concurrently throughout the interviewing period. Following each interview, memos were written, interviews were coded, content analysis was performed, and categories were developed.

Three major categories emerged early in the study:

(1) Learning to touch.
(2) Response to touch.
(3) Touch/talk.

These categories were further analysed after the second interviews using grounded theory concepts outlined by Glaser (1978). These categories became the basis for exploration in succeeding interviews, and they were revised and verified based on feedback from the informants.

Results

The concept of touch

The findings of this study are indicative of the inadequacies of defining touch as skin-to-skin contact. The informants were unable to offer a single definition of touch. 'There are some words you can define and there are some words you can only describe – and that's touch'. Rather, touch was described by the informants as multi-dimensional; a gestalt involving voice, posture, effect, intent and meaning within a context, as well as tactile contact. An understanding of this touch gestalt is dependent on the individual dimensions considered as an integrated cluster. The dimensions of voice, posture (the manner in which the toucher holds and presents his or her body during tactile content), and effect (the subjective impression that posture creates, for instance, eagerness or flatness) are potentially identifiable by observation, as is tactile contact. However, contextually bound meaning and intent, particularly the latter, reside within the nurse as unobservable phenomena. The informants suggested that because of this, it may be impossible to differentiate between different types of touch (e.g. caring touch), or between combined touches, such as when the nurse is combining comforting touch with procedural touch in order to achieve a therapeutic benefit (e.g. decreasing the discomfort of a procedure).

An obvious gap in this conceptualization of touch is the patient's perception. In the ICU, these nurses frequently work with patients whose communicative abilities are severely disrupted. One of the consequences is the frequent assumption that the patient would want to be touched. An examination of the perceptions of nurses who do not incorporate touch into their practice or believe that it is of no potential therapeutic value would add to an understanding of the touch gestalt, as would the inclusion of the patients' perceptions.

Acquiring a touching style

A nurse's touching style is learned. Informants reported that learning occurred during three stages: from their cultural background, while in nursing school, and while working from constant interaction, or feedback from patients (Fig. 6.1). Although there is a temporal ordering to these

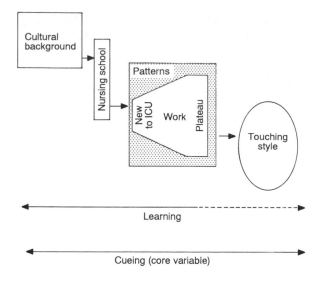

Fig. 6.1   Acquiring a touching style.

stages, they do not stand in isolation; rather they form a matrix that is woven throughout a lifetime of social interaction. Also implicit in this model are the maturation process of the individual as a person and as a nurse, the inter-personal context of the interaction, and the cultural context of the interaction (the norms or patterns of touching of a given subculture). Situational variables or patterns of touch exert an influence on touching style, but they are context bound, temporary, and do not alter the fundamental touching style of a nurse.

Cultural background

Cultural background consists of a composite of the life experiences of the individual nurse, her socialization as a person, and the broader cultural beliefs and norms that she has internalized. As such, it includes her family, education, religion, socio-economic status, and culture, social and personal experiences. The elements of cultural background identified by the infor-mants as the most significant in learning to touch were family, 'street' learning, and personal (one-to-one) experience.

Family

The fundamental association that individuals made with touch, whether sexual, comforting, loving, punitive or depriving, were established in the family origin. People learn to touch within their family by observing, experiencing and cueing (largely non-verbally), in short, by virtue of being present and internalizing the normative patterns of touching for that particular family unit. If the family is a 'touchy' family, with much warm and loving touch, then the children learn to be comfortable with touch and to incorporate touch as a part of their unconscious behaviour. Conversely, if the family is not 'touchy', with little or no warm and loving touch, the members of the family do not learn to be comfortable, and may learn to be uncomfortable with touch. Those that came from 'non-touchy' families attributed less importance in determining touching styles to the family than did those who learned to be comfortable with touch at home. Informants indicated that the uneasiness one had with touching could be countered by actively working at touching and by learning from other situations.

Informants reported that the values that people absorb in the family influence their later touching style. For example, learning to respect the elderly as a child and a young adult can carry over into the nurse's practice in the form of respectful and caring touching with elderly patients. Informants stated that they also learned in their family of attachment. This took the form of increased comfort with touch (both given and receiving), learned from their partners and, for some, from their children. It seems likely that the converse is also true; that is, one could learn discomfort with the use of touch if the relationship was destructive.

Street learning

'Street learning' is the process by which people learn the socially acceptable norms of touch from outside the family and by which they experiment, using trial and error responses (own and others), to touch. As children, adolescents and young adults, people give and receive not only non-verbal but verbal cues, testing in part the cues learned in the family. The sexualizing of touch becomes more clearly identifiable in this phase of learning. Girls learn that touching other girls is at first acceptable and, later, less acceptable. They learn that touching boys is sexually charged. They learn that touch rarely connotes simply comfort in our culture, but rather is laden with implicit sexual meaning. Negative cues are learned in this phase and were clearly remembered by informants. By the later years, an established pattern is set, and the individual feels less need to identify and learn the societal norms.

Personal experience

Personal experience learning refers to the defined touching experiences that individuals have that serve to alter their touching behaviours. For example, one informant described receiving a facial massage (a new experience for her), which she experienced as relaxing and pleasant. She then incorporated this new knowledge into her nursing practice. Similar transference was described with such experiences as foot massages and back rubs. Any new touch experience carries with it the potential for increasing the nurse's awareness of how it feels to be touched and, based on this, the possibility exists for it to be incorporated into her practice. It also seems that the reaction to one's close family and friends to new touch experiences serves a similar function.

Cultural background is a complex stage in learning to touch and acquiring a touching style. It continues throughout one's life, but it seems to be most intense, at least in relation to touch, in childhood, adolescence and young adulthood. Although it is not the sole determinant of a touching style, it is one of the most significant avenues of learning.

Nursing school

Nursing school stands as a separate stage in the learning process because it demarks professional socialization into nursing. As such, it is the first opportunity that the individual has in which to learn about touch as a nursing strategy. Even so, most informants in this study stated that they could recall no explicit reference to touch during their nursing education nor did they believe that their nursing education had indirectly helped them to learn touching behaviours. One informant stated that learning about 'therapeutic communication' had allowed her to transfer some of those principles to touching. All of the informants stated that they should have been taught about touching in nursing school and that structured learning experiences (e.g. workshops) were one way to learn about touch. They also described the process of participating in the research study as one way in which they thought to learn more about touch.

Work

The work phase is the most intense stage of learning about touch specific to nursing, although the learning that occurs is not restricted to nursing practice and is also incorporated into one's private life. It is in the work phase that the nurse becomes enculturated as a nurse and internalizes behavioural norms. In the 'new-to-ICU' phase, the nurse is so overwhelmed by the actual environment, and by the knowledge and technical skills that must be mastered, that she probably does not learn much about touch. She does, however, accumulate the beginning repertoire of ICU beliefs which influences her touching style.

As the nurse moves out of the 'new-to-ICU' phase, she is better able to learn. She begins to listen, to observe role models, and to place herself 'in the patient's shoes'. She rapidly identifies nurses whom she wishes to emulate and learns intensively from them. This learning includes how these nurses interact with patients and how they touch them. Although the informants explained this process, they could not recall ever explicitly thinking 'that nurse is touching in a way that I will try'. Rather, it was the total behaviour of the ideal nurse, of which touch was a part, that they sought to adopt.

After a period of time, learning 'plateaus' and is diminished. During this period, the nurse becomes comfortable in the ICU setting. This appears to be critical to one's ability to use touch effectively. She now becomes susceptible to the effects of routine and boredom, which are for many more difficult to cope with than the daily suffering one encounters in ICU. Boredom adversely affects one's energy level and therefore one's willingness and ability to touch. At this point, cueing, which has been an active mechanism all along, becomes the dominant mechanism by which ICU nurses learn how to touch the individual patient. That is, from this point on, learning about touch is directed more toward learning about the individual patient than it is about touch in general. By this time, the nurse has developed a basic touching style. Any changes in this style are likely to be a result of either the individual nurse's interpersonal experience or a meaningful formal educational event.

Acquiring a touching style, then, is a basic process within which are interwoven other processes and variables that work together in inter-relationship to form the matrix of dynamics that constitute touching style. Although the 'style' of any given nurse is probably established quite early in her working life, as the nurse matures this style will likely also mature.

The core variable

Cuing was identified as the core variable and defined as 'the process by which, through symbolic interaction with others, one determines the need for and the appropriateness of touch, and anticipates the response to, and evaluates the effect of touch'. Cueing is a life-long learning process that is culturally mediated, and it has both personal and professional dimensions; it is critical to understanding the process of touch.

Cueing depends on an individual's ability and willingness to interpret verbal cues and/or the non-verbal cues (such as posture, effect, eye contact and facial expression) of body language. As indicated in Fig. 6.2, cues may be positive or negative.

Non-verbal cues dominate the professional (nursing) sphere, especially in the ICU where most patients are so critically ill that cues are diminished and often subtle. Although cues come predominantly from patients when the nurse initiates the interaction, sometimes cues are given to the patient, especially if the nurse is establishing distance between herself and the patient. In the absence of an ability to cue (e.g. from the pavulonized patient), nurses who use touch therapeutically frequently assume that touch is appropriate, desirable, will be positively received, and be of benefit to the patient.

For the nurse, the most inhibiting response is the patient's negative cue, whether it be verbal or non-verbal, and the most desired cue is the overtly

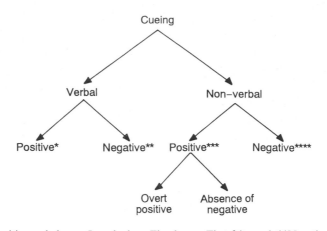

Fig. 6.2 Cueing. *Positive verbal cues: I need a hug, Thank-you, That felt good. **Negative verbal cues: Don't touch me, I'd rather not be touched. ***Positive non-verbal cues: Smiling, Eye contact, Reaching out with hand, Turning toward the nurse, Open facial expression, Leaning toward the nurse, Groping for the nurse, Squeezing nurse's hand, Patient calms after being touched. ****Negative non-verbal cues: Patient withdraws or turns away from nurse's touch, Patient huddles under the linen, Patient swings at or strikes nurse, Patient clenches fists or tightens body posture, Patient folds arms across chest, Patient frowns, Patient stiffens or tightens up, Patient refuses to make eye contact or closes eyes, Patient pushes nurse's hand away, Patient brings knees up to chest.

positive one. It is interesting to note that these informants described the absence of a negative cue as being as strong an indicator as an overtly positive cue. This is probably a reflection of the fact that in ICU many patients cannot cue because they are either unconscious or too encumbered by the therapies of the area (e.g. ventilators, artificial airways, multiple lines and/or medications), and, consequently, nurses become accustomed to receiving no response. Further, these informants indicated that if one believes that touch is a therapeutic tool, then nurses assume that the patient desires to be touched, particularly since they themselves would want to be touched if they were in a similar situation.

The touching process

Entering

The touching process is composed of two stages: entering and connecting (see Fig. 6.3). Entering is the process by which the nurse gains permission to enter the patient's personal space, which the informants referred to as the patient's 'bubble' or boundary. This bubble is the delineated area surrounding individuals and protecting them from the inappropriate violation of self.

To enter this personal space, the nurse uses talking. This talking phase serves two purposes: it warns the patient that the nurse is making an overture to enter, described by one informant as 'cueing him up', and it permits the

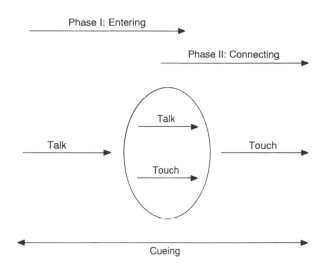

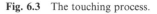

Fig. 6.3 The touching process.

nurse to obtain information about the patient's need for, probable response to, and the propriety of being touched. Even if the patient is intubated and unable to speak but alert and able to respond by shaking his or her head and using non-verbal language, the nurse uses talk, and non-verbal patient cues become paramount. If the patient is non-responsive, disturbances occur, because the nurse is unsure whether or not the patient is warned or what the patient's probable response will be to touch. Interestingly, the absence of a patient's cue does not always result in skipping this phase; rather, nurses seem to continue to go through the motions of entering out of habit and because of the commonly held belief that even unresponsive patients may be able to hear.

Once the nurse has obtained permission (consent) to enter, the next phase is one of both talking and touching. Actively seeking permission to enter and touch continues, and the nurse is now committed to a closer relationship with the patient. As she moves into the more intimate space zones, she is increasingly at risk of being rejected. Consequently, there is more active, complex and sensitive cueing occurring as the nurse tries to establish a 'connection' with the patient. The nurse has now made a commitment to interacting meaningfully with the patient and to expending the emotional energy required to connect with the patient.

Connecting

The touch/talk phase now intensifies, and the nurse moves into the connecting stage which is frequently characterized by reciprocity, although this reciprocity may be subtle and not easily identifiable. Connecting is a highly individualized and complex process whereby the nurse allows herself to care about the patient. This places the ICU nurse in a position of being vulnerable to feeling and to caring about the patient's well-being. The feelings may be those of satisfaction, reward or joy if the patient does well, or they may be the less desirable feelings of emotional pain, sorrow, anger or grief if the patient does not do well.

As nurses in ICU are constantly barraged with human tragedies, they are cautious about exposing themselves to the potentially draining emotions that can result from this process. The final phase of connecting is touching, which is more than, but includes, skin-to-skin contact. It is in this phase that the touching process is completed. One informant described this completion of the touching process as 'bumping souls'.

Informants said that there were any possible number of 'infractions' in this process of touching. For instance, the nurse may go directly to an intimate touch without warning the patient or may go through the motions of seeking permission to enter their personal space with no real intent of actually obtaining or using the information received from the cueing process. Alternatively, the nurse can ignore the process all together, especially if touch is not in her repertoire of therapeutic strategies. Any of these infractions can more easily occur with the non-responsive patient who is unable to participate in the process. Moreover, the informants stated a belief that the ICU patient's and, particularly, the non-responsive ICU patient's personal space has a different configuration from that of non-patients. Terms such as 'shrinking' were used to describe what was perceived to be a permeable, altered boundary that no longer ensured integrity of personal space. From their personal lives, nurses are acutely aware of their feelings and the reactions of others to boundary violations and to the inappropriate use of touch. In touching patients, the informants indicated that a significant component of the propriety of touch is related to patient consent.

Discussion

The touch gestalt

Although Weiss did not describe its constituent elements, in 1979 she discussed a 'tactile gestalt'. Implicit evidence that the elements identified in this study are integral to touch can be found in the literature. In their assessment of the effects of touch, some investigators have used non-verbal indicators such as facial expression, eye contact and body movement as measures of the effect of touch (Knable, 1981; Langland & Panicucci, 1982; McCorkle, 1974). Montagu refers to 'emotion, feeling, affect, and touch' as 'scarcely separable from one another' (1986). Weiss's (1979, 1986) and

Pepler's (1984) theoretical frameworks incorporate multiple dimensions of the touch experience; and meaning and context as critical elements of a touch gestalt are supported by the work of Morse (1983) and Jones & Yarbrough (1985).

Inherent in the traditional definitions of touch is the basic assumption that touch is a phenomenon that is appropriately defined (operationally) as skin-to-skin contact. This implies that touch is observable and measurable, and that there is, as Weiss (1986) has stated, 'an assumption that all types of touch carry the same meaning'. The result has been an extremely narrow definition of touch which has fundamentally influenced research design and measurement. This definition of touch, and its failure to include the 'other than physical' dimensions of touch, constitutes the main threat to the validity of existing research on touch; that is, there is no research base to support the theoretical supposition that touch can be adequately defined as skin-to-skin contact. In fact, this study's findings show that there is support for the consideration of multiple dimensions in any type of touch and for further examination to elicit a more complete theoretical model of the gestalt of touch.

Cueing

Cueing as a process integral to touching has not been previously reported. However, studies that report using verbal and, particularly, non-verbal behaviours, such as facial expression, eye contact and body movement (Knable, 1981; Langland & Panicucci, 1982; McCorkle, 1974), suggest that these behaviours are 'cues' in the effective use of touch. Two studies on nursing intuition discuss the use of 'cues'. Young (1987) states: 'Cues represent the information that the nurses used to make a decision and range from subjective feeling cues to objective physical signs'. Schraeder & Fischer (1987) identify perception of cues by nurses as one of four factors in intuitive knowledge. From these two sources, the following inferences can be drawn:

(1) There is support for the validity of the cues identified in this study.
(2) The identification of cues (i.e. cueing) may be a more general and pervasive process than is presently recognized, that is, not limited to touching.
(3) Intuitive knowledge and decision-making may be only one dimension of cueing.

One question that must be raised in relation to cueing is the impact of the patient's cultural background on the nurses' ability accurately to identify and interpret patients' cues. Do different cultures assign different meanings to cues or, in fact, give such different cues that the nurse must understand cultural variation in cueing, or are there universally understood cues in relation to touching?

Proxemic considerations

Personal space is an intrinsic dimension of the touching process. Informants were acutely aware of patients' personal space, which they often referred to as a 'bubble' or boundary. These findings are consistent with the proxemic literature (Hayduk, 1983). The aspects of the touching model (Fig. 6.3) that are particularly relevant to patient proxemics, and which have implications for practice, are the issues of permission or consent to enter and the suggestion that the personal space of ICU patients may 'shrink' or change in some manner due to the violative nature of the ICU. Personal space is a significant dimension of the touching process and this literature could be a fruitful source of information in considering the model's further development.

Learning to touch

The process by which nurses (or people) learn to touch has not previously been described. There is support for culture as a major influence, but specific cultural dimensions have not been described. Weiss alludes to the family of origin as a significant influence (1990) and expands on this in later work (1992). The mechanisms the informants described using in the work phase (role modelling, observing, listening, putting self 'in patient's shoes') were learned non-verbally by 'osmosis'. This is similar to aspects of the intuition studies cited earlier and to the work of Benner (1984). It seems plausible that such 'informal' learning is the primary mechanism by which nurses learn to use touch in their practice. As such, it would have implications for the manner in which nurses are taught clinically, both as students and as graduates. Exemplar role models appear to be able to exert a powerful and lasting influence on nurses.

Conclusions

These findings add substantively to a beginning understanding of how nurses touch. An understanding of the mechanisms of touch is critical to our ability to recognize both inappropriate and context appropriate deviation from a norm. An understanding of how nurses learn to touch and acquire a touching style is required if we are to act on observed deviations in the touching process or teach the appropriate use of touch. If touching is a primitive and potent human act, if touching is central to nursing practice, and if its effects can be positive, neutral or negative, then it is essential that the mechanisms of touch be understood.

It is particularly important if we are to begin to develop strategies that will be useful additions to nursing curricula and to clinical and classroom teaching contexts. It is disturbing that the informants in this study reported that explicit material on touch had not been present in their nursing education. There is no support for an assumption that students are adequately equipped to incorporate contextually appropriate touch into their practice either as a therapeutic nursing strategy, or as a non-harmful incidental. Although, to adequately incorporate material on touch into educational contexts requires a much more thorough understanding than is presently available, studies such as this offer beginning insights into the many dimensions that require explication. They also enable us to begin active reconsideration of touch in both our own and our students' practices, and to incorporate these beginning descriptions of the ways in which nurses learn to touch into our understanding of why disturbances appear in the practice of some. This understanding will assist as we begin to reflect on how to help nurses and nursing students enhance their therapeutic use of touch.

Bottorff (1991), in her critical review of the research on nurse–patient touch, identified the salient methodological problems found within this research. She supports the need for further inductive work in the area in order for theory development to proceed. Such theoretical work will result in more fruitful deductive work. Several of the findings in this study have not been previously reported or discussed in the literature, so the question must be raised. How do they contribute to existing knowledge on touch?

First, they provide new insights by interviewing the nurse whose perspective has been largely omitted from previous investigation on touch. Second, the findings have the potential to contribute to the development of a theory of touch by adding to existing work in nursing on touch, namely that of Weiss (1979, 1986) and Pepler (1984). Third, the findings of this study reinforce the value of systematically examining behaviours that have been taken for granted because they are so much a part of everyday practice and seeming common sense.

Further investigation

Questions have been raised that merit further investigation: Under what conditions does the touching process described hold? Is there a different configuration in the personal space of ICU patients? If so, what is it and what implications are there for nurses? Can touch be effectively taught in nursing schools? What methods are best suited to this? How does the nurse's cultural learning about touch, acquired prior to entering nursing, affect subsequent learning? Are there other ways in which nurses learn to cue? How do nurses validate their cues? Can cuing be taught? Answers to these questions and to others that will arise from them will assist us in understanding the therapeutic use of touch in our practice.

Acknowledgements

The authors wish to acknowledge Dr Marion Allen and Dr Norah Keating for their advice and support. Financial support was provided by a National Health Research Development Programme (NHRDP) Fellowship, by a Canadian Nurses' Foundation award to C. Estabrooks, and an NHRDP Research Scholar award to Dr J. Morse. This chapter is based on Ms Estabrooks' master's thesis (1987) completed at the University of Alberta, Edmonton, under the supervision of Dr Janice Morse.

References

Barnett, K.A. (1972) A survey of the current utilization of touch by health team personnel with hospitalized patients. *International Journal of Nursing Studies*, **9**, 195–209.

Benner, P. (1984) *From Novice to Expert: Excellence and Power in Clinical Nursing Practice.* Addison-Wesley, Don Mills, Ontario.

Birch, E.R. (1986) The experience of touch received during labor. *Journal of Nurse–Midwifery*, **31**, 270–75.

Bottorff, J.L. (1991) A methodological review and evaluation of research on nurse–patient touch. In *Anthology on Caring* (ed. P.L. Chinn), pp. 303–43. National League for Nursing Press, New York.

Bottorff, J.L. (1992) Nurse–patient interaction: Observations of touch. Doctoral dissertation, University of Alberta. *Dissertation Abstracts International*, **53** (12), 6217–B.

Burnside, I.M. (1981) The therapeutic use of touch. In *Nursing and the Aged* (ed. I.M. Burnside) pp. 503–18. McGraw-Hill, Toronto.

Clement, J.M. (1983) A descriptive study of the use of touch by nurses with patients in the critical-care unit. Doctoral dissertation, the University of Texas at Austin. *Dissertation Abstracts International*, **43**, 1060B.

Clement, J.M. (1987) Touch: research findings and use in preoperative care. *AORN Journal*, **45**, 1429–39.

DeWever, M.K. (1977) Nursing home patients' perception of nurses' affective touch. *The Journal of Psychology*, **96**, 163–71.

El-Kafass, A.A.R. (1983) A study of expressive touch behaviours by nursing personnel with patients in critical care units. Doctoral dissertation, the Catholic University of America. *Dissertation Abstracts International*, **43**, 3187B.

Estabrooks, C.A. (1987) Touch in nursing practice: a historical perspective. *Journal of Nursing History*, **2**(2), 33–49.

Estabrooks, C.A. (1989). Touch: a nursing strategy in the ICU. *Heart & Lung*, **18**, 391–401.

Glaser, B.G. (1978) *Theoretical Sensitivity*. The Sociology Press, Mill Valley, California.

Glaser, B.G. & Strauss, A.L. (1967) *The Discovery of Grounded Theory*. Aldine Publishing, New York.

Glick, M.S. (1986) Caring touch and anxiety in myocardial infarction patients in the intermediate cardiac care unit. *Intensive Care Nursing*, **2**, 61–6.

Hayduk, L.A. (1983) Personal space: where we now stand. *Psychological Bulletin*, **94**, 293–335.

Jones, S.E. & Yarbrough, A.E. (1985) A naturalistic study of the meanings of touch. *Communication Monographs*, **52**, 19–56.

Knable, J. (1981) Handholding: one means of transcending barriers of communication. *Heart & Lung*, **10**, 1106–10.

Krieger, D. (1975) Therapeutic touch: the imprimatur of nursing. *The American Journal of Nursing*, **8**, 152–5.

Langland, R.M. & Panicucci, C.L. (1982) Effects of touch on communication with elderly confused clients. *Journal of Gerontological Nursing*, **8**, 152–5.

McCorkle, R. (1974) Effects of touch on seriously ill patients. *Nursing Research*, **23**, 125–32.

Mitchell, P.H., Habermann-Little, B., Johnson, F., Vanlnwegen-Scott, D. & Tyler, D. (1985) Critically ill children: the importance of touch in a high technology environment. *Nursing Administration Quarterly*, **9**, 38–46.

Montagu, A. (1986) *Touching: The Human Significance of the Skin*, 3rd edn. Harper & Row, New York.

Morse, J.M. (1983) An ethnoscientific analysis of comfort: a preliminary investigation. *Nursing Papers*, **15**, 6–19.

Penny, K.S. (1979) Postpartum perception of touch received during labor. *Research in Nursing and Health*, **2**, 9–16.

Pepler, C.J. (1984) Congruence in relational messages communicated to nursing home residents through nurse aide touch behaviours. Doctoral dissertation. The University of Michigan, 1984. *Dissertation Abstracts International*, **45**, 2106B.

Porter, L., Redfern, S., Wilson-Barnett, J. & LeMay, A. (1986) The development of an observation schedule for measuring nurse–patient touch, using an ergonomic approach. *International Journal of Nursing Studies*, **23**, 11–20.

Schraeder, B.D. & Fischer, D.K. (1987) Using intuitive knowledge in the neonatal intensive care nursery. *Holistic Nursing Practice*, **1**(3), 45–51.

Watson, W.H. (1975) The meanings of touch: geriatric nursing. *Journal of Communication*, **25**, 104–12.

Weiss, S.J. (1979). The language of touch. *Nursing Research*, **28**, 76–80.

Weiss, S.J. (1986) Psychophysiologic effects of caregiver touch on incidence of cardiac dysrhythmia. *Heart & Lung*, **15**, 495–505.

Weiss, S.J. (1990) Effects of differential touch on nervous system arousal of patients recovering from cardiac disease. *Heart & Lung*, **19**, 474–80.

Weiss, S.J. (1992) Measurement of the sensory qualities in tactile interaction. *Nursing Research*, **41**, 82–6.

Young, C.E. (1987) Intuition and the nursing process. *Holistic Nursing Practice*, **1**(3), 52–62.

Chapter 7
Can combined oral contraceptives be made more effective by means of a nursing care model?

MARIANNE LINDELL, *BSc(Nursing and Midwifery)*,
UD in Nursing Education
Doctoral Student/research assistant

and HENNY OLSSON, *PhD, BSc, BSc(Nursing, Midwifery and Public Health Nursing), UD in Nursing Education*
Professor pro tem, Research Supervisor, Center for Caring Sciences, Örebro Medical Center Hospital, Örebro, Sweden

This chapter is a theoretical attempt to show how the Neuman Systems Model can be practically used in combined oral contraceptive counselling by Swedish midwives. Counselling regarding combined oral contraceptives is not solely of a medical nature. There are many dimensions of care, namely sociological, developmental and philosophical. In 1980, the midwife in Sweden was responsible for between 70–80% of counselling in contraceptive methods. To facilitate the contraceptive counselling by the midwives, the Neuman Systems Model can be used as a theoretical aid. In the present report, the midwife's oral contraceptive counselling is described at an individual level with primary prevention. It is concluded that, from a theoretical standpoint, it is not possible to predict how the Neuman Systems Model, as a theoretical aid for the midwife, can increase the effectiveness of the birth control pill in preventing pregnancy. Research about the use of the nursing care model in oral contraceptive counselling should be carried out.

Introduction

This chapter is a theoretical attempt to show how Betty Neuman's nursing care model (Neuman 1982) can be practically used in combined oral contraceptive counselling provided by Swedish midwives.

A nursing care model can be an aid for the midwife in structuring counselling in the use of combined oral contraceptives. Advice concerning combined oral contraceptives is not solely of a medical character. There are a number of dimensions of care, namely sociological, physiological, developmental and philosophical. Neuman's Systems Model would be expected to be suitable, since the goal of the model is to help the caregiver focus, identify and, above all, give a preventive perspective, i.e. to prevent stress factors.

Preventive nursing care can take place at three different levels: primary, secondary and tertiary. The model can be used at community, organizational and individual levels. The midwife's work in family planning, the purpose of which is to avoid unwanted pregnancy, takes place at the individual level within primary prevention. When she is providing counselling, the midwife must be clear about prevention, stressors and reactions which are relevant in this context, in order for the model to be functionally applicable. To be able to prescribe birth-control pills, the midwife must have complex professional skills through which she can increase the woman's awareness about the effects of the pills.

Purpose

This chapter aims to explore how the Swedish midwife can use the Neuman Systems Model practically in providing combined oral contraceptive counselling.

Background

During the past few years, the frequency of legal abortions in Sweden has increased. There is no sign of any decrease; rather the tendency is toward an additional increase. The increase in abortion is most marked in women under the age of 25 years. A modest increase can be observed among older women. Abortions among teenagers in Sweden are increasing after a declining trend at the end of the 1970s and beginning of the 1980s. (For the years 1975 and 1983 there were 23.8 and 25.2 legal abortions/100 pregnancies respectively.) In the teenage group, legal abortions are increasing most among the 17–18-year-olds (National Swedish Board of Health and Welfare, 1988). Table 7.1 shows the distribution of abortions within different age groups during the years 1987 and 1988 (preliminary data) (National Swedish Board of Health and Welfare, 1989).

When a new abortion law came into effect in 1975, the Swedish Parliament resolved that great attention would be given to measures which could prevent the need for abortions. Sweden's capacity for providing contraceptive counselling is now good (Statistics of the National Swedish Board of Health and Welfare, 1984).

In Sweden, sixty per cent of all women between the ages of 20 and 44 years use some form of birth control (Statistics of the National Swedish Board of Health and Welfare, 1982). Of the available contraceptive measures, the

Table 7.1   Abortions performed in 1987 and 1988 divided into 5-year age groups and per 1000 women in the respective age groups.

Age	1987			1988		
	n	%	Per 1000 women	*n*	%	Per 1000 women
Up to 19	5874	17.0	21.4	6614	17.7	24.2
20–24	9273	26.9	30.7	10161	27.3	33.5
25–29	6655	19.3	24.4	7345	19.7	26.5
30–34	5338	15.5	18.9	5750	15.4	20.3
35–39	4749	13.8	15.7	4667	12.5	15.9
40 and over	2596	7.5	8.0	2730	7.3	8.3
Unknown				7		
Totals	34486	100	19.6	37275	100	21.2

Table 7.2   Contraceptive methods used by women in different age groups (in percentages).

	20–24	25–29	30–34	35–39	40–44
Natural methods	4	7	7	11	12
Barrier methods	23	28	33	38	45
Oral contraceptives	61	37	25	20	15
Intrauterine devices	12	28	35	31	28

birth-control pill is the most effective protection against unwanted pregnancy. It is also the contraceptive method used by most women in Sweden, about one-third of all users (Statistics of the National Swedish Board of Health and Welfare, 1982). Table 7.2 shows the distribution of contraceptive methods for women in the different age groups.

The anticonceptive oral hormone combination preparations contain oestrogen and progesterone and are taken daily for 21–22 days, followed by seven or six pill-free days, respectively (National Swedish Board of Health and Welfare, 1987). The combination preparation inhibits growth of the follicle, ovulation, cervical secretion and growth of the endometrium. It is almost 100% effective, provided that pills are taken correctly. In practice, however, there is between 0.1 and 1 pregnancy per 100 women due to incorrect use of the pills.

When treatment is first begun, there can be side-effects such as slight nausea, weight gain, breast tenderness, depression and decreased libido. As a rule, menstruation decreases and after long-term use bleeding can also occur (so-called spotting). A moderate increase in blood pressure has been seen and there is some risk of deep vein thrombosis. The blood pressure almost always decreases when oral contraceptives are discontinued.

Studies show that there is some risk of cardiovascular disease in women aged 40–44 years, although smoking is a greater risk factor than the use of oral contraceptives. Some effect on the liver and general itchiness and jaundice have been reported. Gall bladder symptoms occur more often in women using birth-control pills. In regard to reproductive organ tumours, epidemiological studies have shown that combination birth-control pills are associated with a significantly lower risk for endometrial cancer during use and also after the pills have been discontinued. Epidemiological studies are contradictory concerning the relation between use of birth-control pills and breast cancer (National Swedish Board of Health and Welfare, 1987).

Counselling

Counselling on contraception and information about preventing the need for abortion constitute part of the preventive health care which county councils are by law required to provide. A great deal of such counselling is offered via maternity health care. In 1980, the percentage of such counselling provided by the midwife was between 70–80% in almost all counties (Swedish Government Official Reports, 1983).

In her role within maternity health care, the Swedish midwife is called upon to act as a counsellor. In addition to other functions, midwives with a specific degree in anticonception are to provide the medical service necessary so that modern methods of contraception can be used. Such counselling can comprise information and discussion about different methods of birth control, gynaecological examinations to assess the size and position of the uterus, and, in normal cases, the insertion of an intrauterine contraceptive device (IU(C)D) or preparations for prescribing birth-control pills. Special office hours must be set aside for counselling. Time must also be allotted for telephone counselling and information directed towards the public. Midwives give contraceptive advice to those who want it during the postpartum examination (National Swedish Board of Health and Welfare, 1979).

The Neuman Systems Model

The Neuman Systems Model (Neuman 1982) is a systems model which views the patient from a holistic perspective. Neuman schematically describes her system of four circles encircling one another. All the circles work together. The innermost circle is called the core and comprises the ego, genetic structure and physiologically important life functions. The next circle after the core is designated by Neuman as the individual's basic defence. Then the model shows the individual's normal line of defence, which has some stability in contrast to the fourth and outermost circle, which is flexible.

Neuman works with three categories of stressors which can affect the individual's reactions and behaviour. By stressors, she means different

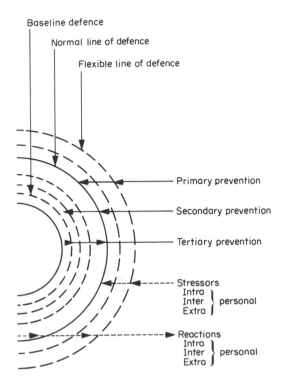

Baseline defence

Normal line of defence

Flexible line of defence

Primary prevention

Secondary prevention

Tertiary prevention

Stressors
Intra ⎫
Inter ⎬ personal
Extra ⎭

Reactions
Intra ⎫
Inter ⎬ personal
Extra ⎭

Fig. 7.1   The Neuman systems model for nursing care adapted for the individual level by Lindell & Olsson (Neuman (1982). (Used with permission.)

factors which are interpreted as threats within or outside the person and which can affect his reactions and behaviour.

According to Neuman, the goal of the theoretical working model is to help the caregiver by identifying the stressors in the patient and, with the help of the patient, to make her conscious of and prepared to react to stressors so that balance is maintained within the system.

Intervention can take place at three different levels:

(1) Primary prevention: the intervention is preventive, that is precedes any reaction to stressors. The caregiver helps the person strengthen her flexible line of defence.
(2) Secondary prevention: the caregiver intervenes after symptoms have arisen.
(3) Tertiary prevention: occurs when one or more stressors threaten the core and all available resources must be used to maintain balance in the system.

Neuman's model can be used at community, institutional and individual levels (Neuman, 1982; Carpers *et al.*, 1985; Gavan *et al.*, 1988).

Limitations

The midwife uses Neuman's model for primary prevention at the individual level when providing counselling concerning the combination of oral contraceptives at the woman's first visit to the clinic.

Application of the model to counselling

In Neuman's model, the midwife's combined oral contraceptive counselling comprises primary prevention at the individual level. The goal of primary prevention in combined oral contraceptive counselling is to prevent risks that a stressor will threaten the core, that is, unwanted pregnancy, and to strengthen the flexible line of defence. Preventive actions consist of clarifying for the woman what a stressor is. The midwife is supposed to give the woman verbal and written information about the combined oral contraceptives and their use. The midwife should use the stress factors positively in her preventive work.

According to Neuman's model, the woman's psyche and soma can be likened to a system, and an unwanted pregnancy is the stressor which threatens the core (core, threat to the woman's ego).

Examples are given below of the different variables and stressors at individual level which can affect the woman's use of oral contraceptives; primary prevention is required.

Sociocultural variables

Availability for an appointment for combined oral contraceptive counselling can be reduced due to difficulties the woman may have co-ordinating her work hours or studies with the midwife's office hours. Geographical difficulties in coming to the office can also decrease availability, as can economic circumstances.

Psychological variables

Knowledge about the absence of ovulation can influence how the woman experiences her female identity. Smoking may be considered more important than correct use of the birth-control pills. The effect of information via the mass media can influence motivation. An unconscious psychological stress factor could be expressed in carelessness and forgetting to take the pills.

Physiological variables

Physiological stressors could be unaccepted weight increase. Smoking and age are two factors which should be considered as stressors, since the risk of thrombosis increases. Gastroenteritis and diarrhoea should be considered as strong stressors, which is why a woman suffering from such ailments should use additional means of contraception in addition to combined oral contraceptives.

Philosophical/spiritual variables

Religious and cultural heritage can be a stress factor if it clashes with a woman's view of having children and a career. Ambivalence towards birth-control pills is a risk if uncertainties about what the woman wants cannot be clarified.

Developmental variables

As a rule, intellectual development is somewhat ahead of emotional development in younger age groups. An explanation of how birth-control pills work and their use must be made particularly clear to women in younger-age categories. Consequences for the woman of an unwanted pregnancy must be pointed out in a positive way, irrespective of whether she completes the pregnancy or not. In other words, she must be given support regardless of the decision she makes.

Interpersonal stressors

The relationship between a man and a woman can unconsciously/consciously interfere with the use of the oral contraceptives. For instance, if the woman would prefer not to take birth-control pills and the man does not want to use condoms, the stress factor is significantly increased. Differing ideas and values the pair may have regarding having a baby could interfere with the woman's use of birth-control pills.

Intrapersonal stressors

Intrapersonal stressors include the woman's ambivalence between maintaining a career and having a baby and fear about side-effects from the birth-control pills. Intellectual ability to use information about the oral contraceptives properly may be lacking.

Extrapersonal stressors

Extrapersonal stressors can be present if the personnel providing birth-control counselling are unable to adapt the information to the individual woman's situation. Values and attitudes of persons close to the woman (parents, friends, etc.) about combined oral contraceptives may also have an effect. Information from the mass media which the woman sorts through and reinterprets can jeopardize her use of birth-control pills.

The results of stressors which are not prevented can be demonstrated in terms of the woman's reactions and behaviour. For example, one reaction can be dissatisfaction with the sexual relationship between men and women (no desire, too tired for intercourse). Forgetfulness and carelessness about taking the birth-control pills can be regarded as behaviour indicating an unconscious (not worked through) wish to be pregnant. Pregnancy due to the fact that oral contraception is an unsafe method of birth control when the woman has diarrhoea indicates that the woman did not receive proper information or that she did not understand it.

Importance of the nursing care model

We have indicated that Neuman's model can be used as an aid or theoretical basis for the Swedish midwife when she is providing oral-contraceptive counselling. By helping the woman to prevent different stress factors concerning birth-control pills, the model can be of positive significance both for life in general and for the relationship between women and men.

Conclusion

It is not possible at the present time to predict how the practical application of the model to combined oral contraceptive counselling affects the use of birth-control pills. In order to obtain more information about whether combined oral contraceptive counselling using the nursing care model has any effect (decreasing number of abortions), research in which traditional birth-control counselling is compared with counselling using Neuman's model must be carried out.

References

Carpers, C., Quinn, R., Kelly, R. & Fenerty, A. (1985) The Neuman System Model in practice. *Journal of Nursing Administration*, **15**, 29–39.
Gavan, C., Hastings-Tolsman, M. & Troyan, P. (1988) Explication of Neuman's model: a holistic systems approach to nutrition for health promoting in the life process. *Holistic Nursing Practice*, **3**(1), 26–38.
National Swedish Board of Health and Welfare (1979) *Counselling and Birth Control, 1979:4. Maternity and Childcaring* (Socialstyrelsen redovisar (1979) *Rådgivning och Födelsekontroll 1979: 4. Mödra-och Barnhälsovård.*) Norstedts Tryckeri, Stockholm.

National Swedish Board of Health and Welfare (1987) *Common Advice from the National Swedish Board of Health and Welfare, 1987:6. Anticonception* (Socialstyrelsen (1987) *Allmänna Råd från Socialstyrelsen, 1987:6 Antikonception.*) Allmänna Förlaget AB, Kundtjänst, Stockholm.
National Swedish Board of Health and Welfare (1988) *The Number of Abortion Increases. What Can Be Done to Change the Development?* Preliminary Report About the Situation of Abortion and Preventive Work 1975–1988. (Socialstyrelsen (1988) *Antalet aborter ökar-Vad kan göras för att vända utvecklingen?* Preliminär rapport om abortsituationen och det förebyggande arbetet 1975–1988). Norstedts Tryckeri, Stockholm.
National Swedish Board of Health and Welfare (1989) *Press Communication of the National Swedish Board of Health and Welfare 1989 02 22.* (Socialstyrelsens hälsoupplysningsbyrå (1989) *Pressmeddelande från Socialsytrelsen 1989 02 22.*) Nordstedts Tryckeri, Stockholm.
Neuman, B. (1982) *The Neuman Systems Model. Application to Nursing Education and Practice.* Appleton–Century–Crofts. Norwalk, Connecticut.
Statistics of the National Swedish Board of Health and Welfare (1982) *Women and Children. Interviews With Women About Family and Work, 1982:4.* (Sveriges officiella statistik (1982) *Kvinnor och Barn. Intervjeur Med Kvinnor Om Familj och Arbete. 1982:4.*) Liber Förlag, Stockholm.
Statistics of the National Swedish Board of Health and Welfare (1984) *Free Means Fewer. An Evaluation of the Swedish Abortion Act and Family Planning Programme of 1974. 1984:3* (Sveriges officiella statistik (1984) *Färre Aborter. Svensk Familjeplanering och Abortlag i Ett Internationellt Perspektiv. 1984:3.*) SCB-Tryck, Örebro, Sweden.
Swedish Government Official Reports (1983) *Family Planning and Abortion, 1983:31.* (Statens offentliga utredningar (1983) *Familjeplanering och Abort, 1983:31.*) Minab/Gotab, Stockholm.

Chapter 8
Advice concerning breastfeeding from mothers of infants admitted to a neonatal intensive care unit: the Roy Adaptation Model as a conceptual structure

KERSTIN HEDBERG NYQVIST, *RN, BSN*

Clinical Nurse Specialist, Neonatal Intensive Care Unit 95F, University Hospital

and PER-OLOW SJÖDÉN, *PhD*

Professor, Centre for Caring Sciences, Uppsala University, University Hospital, Uppsala, Sweden

Data were collected by telephone interviews with 178 mothers of full-term patients in a NICU (neonatal intensive care unit) concerning advice on facilitation of the initiation of breastfeeding. The main advice to the first author as a nurse in the NICU concerned the environment, advice on breastfeeding, distance between units, work organization and nurse behaviour. The advice to other mothers of patients centred on persistence, physical contact with the infant, and not to let nurses take over maternal role functions. The data were structured into themes and categories, classified by one author and two research assistants according to Roy's adaptation theory, and analysed for degree of interrater agreement in order to test the operationalization of the theory in an NICU. The overall agreement of classification was high, reaching 92.5%. It was easily applied by nurses after a brief introduction and proved useful for structuring interview data. It also contributed to clarification of nurse behaviour and division of roles between nurses and mothers. As the four adaptation modes showed considerable overlap, this kind of classification seems inadvisable for application to the assessment of patient/parent situations in the nursing process. For use in a clinical setting, the theory needs the addition of the interactive aspect of nurse and patient/family role functions, and may then be used as a framework for the development of assessment tools.

Background

In the spring of 1990, the NICU (neonatal intensive care unit) of the University Hospital in Uppsala, Sweden, adopted an ideology for nursing based

Table 8.1 The four adaptation modes with their respective subheadings according to Callista Roy's adaptation theory.

Physiological needs	Role functions	Self-concept	Interdependence
Oxygen and circulation	Primary roles	Physical self	
Fluids and electrolytes	Secondary roles	Personal self:	
Nutrition	Tertiary roles	self-consistency	
Elimination		self ideal	
Exercise and rest		moral–ethical self	
Protection from pain, inconvenience, heat/cold, damage to the skin			
All the senses: over/ under-stimulation			
Endocrine functions			
Neurological functions			

on Sister Callista Roy's adaptation theory (Roy, 1980; Roy & Roberts, 1981). The ideology was formulated deductively and consists of a description of the nursing activities in an NICU based on the four adaptation modes: physiological needs, role functions, self-concept and interdependence (Table 8.1). According to Roy, some of the main foci of nursing research are life situations where positive (adaptative) processes are threatened by health technology and behavioural problems. When an infant is transferred to an NICU, one particular expression of the relation between mother and child – breastfeeding – is likely to be influenced by routines in neonatal care. In addition, breastfeeding can be conveniently studied.

The focus of the present study is comments and advice given by the patients' mothers on the facilitation of breastfeeding initiation. The purpose is to test the interrater agreement in classification of mothers' comments and advice, and to structure and interpret this information according to the theory as an attempt at operationalization and interpretation of the theory in the NICU setting.

Review of the literature

In the paediatric setting, the adaptation theory can serve as a structure for individual care plans covering all aspects of the situation of the child and its family (Galligan, 1979). Roy (1980; Roy & Roberts, 1981) describes nursing activities as the identification of stimuli leading to adaptative or maladaptative behaviour, both physiologically and psychosocially. Thus, the theory is well suited to paediatric intensive care where the identification of stress factors in children (Munn & Tichy, 1987) and parents (Miles & Carter, 1983) is mandatory. It also provides a theoretical framework for the evaluation of nursing activities in neonatal intensive care using physiological parameters (Norris *et al.*, 1982).

In the intensive care setting, a particular strength of the theory lies in the fact that it does not limit assessment of patients' needs merely to physiological processes and negative behaviour (symptoms). Instead, the assessment should include influential factors in the patient's background and life situation as well as the interaction between persons and their environment. It assists in identifying and stressing positive stimuli and behaviours that can contribute to recovery (Hamner, 1989). It has also been found useful as a framework for a pre-operative assessment tool for post-anaesthesia care unit nurses (Jackson, 1990).

The paucity of reported research that specifically tests nursing theories has been suggested as a deterrent to the development of the scientific base for nursing. The reason for this paucity may be a lack of clarity about what constitutes testing of nursing theories, a question currently under debate. A common approach has focused on determining the validity of a theory by examining the empirical validity of concepts and relational statements and defining criteria for evaluation (Silva, 1986; Acton *et al.*, 1991). Recently approaches other than empirical testing have been proposed in order to reduce the dogma associated with logical positivism, and currently the situation is rather one of plurality than consensus about methods for testing theories (Silva & Sorrel, 1992).

Problem

A problem in testing the theory is the distinction between the three psychosocial modes (role functions, self-concept and interdependence), as they tend to overlap (Wagner, 1976). In the research setting, the theory offers guidance in the design and process of a study, both in the choice of phenomena to be studied, the definition of the problem and in the classification and interpretation of results (Fawcett & Tulman, 1990). In nursing education in Sweden, as well as in other countries, however, there are problems concerning the integration of nursing theory and nursing practice, and among nurses and nurse teachers there is even a concern that theory-based nursing is a threat to the quality of nursing care (Norberg & Wickstrom, 1990).

Method

Sample

The criteria for subject selection were that the infant was a full-term singleton, admitted within his first day of life, discharged within six days, not treated with intensive care (by CPAP, ventilator or total parental nutrition), did not have any congenital malformation or severe disease such as chromosomal abnormality, and that the mother could speak Swedish. All children born in the catchment area of the University Hospital (viz. Uppsala County) during one year, from September 1989 to August 1990, were included. The sample consisted of 178 children, 92 boys and 86 girls, and their mothers, 102 of which were primiparas, 51 were having their second child, and 25 had two or more children before. Ninety-nine of the deliveries were made by Caesarean section – 13 planned and 86 unplanned. Sixty-three of the vaginal deliveries were normal, and 15 were of other types. A majority of the mothers, 82.6%, were given some type of analgesic (80.2% were given pethidine), 87.5% delivered by Caesarian section had full narcosis and the others had epidural or spinal anaesthesia. The mothers' ages ranged from 18 to 42 years, with a mean of 29.1 and a median of 29.

The infants had one or several diagnoses, ranked in the following order of decreasing prevalence: observation after a Caesarian section, low or high birthweight, neonatal distress, hypoglycaemia, maternal diabetes mellitus, fetal distress during labour and neonatal respiratory disturbance. Most of the infants were observed and treated in the NICU for a very short period of time: 29.2% were discharged on the day of admittance and 38.2% on the day after birth. Most of the infants, 74.7% were fed sterilized breastmilk or infant formula, 19.1% were fed by gavage tube one or several times, and 21.3% were given intravenous glucose infusions.

Only ten of the mothers were able to start breastfeeding within the first hour after birth. Forty per cent of the primiparas started breastfeeding on the day of birth or the day after, and very few waited until after three days. Most of the infants, 71.9%, were fully breastfed at discharge from hospital, fewer among the children of primiparas. The proportion of infants who were fully breastfed was higher for those with only one or two days' stay in the NICU. More than half of the children treated for 3–6 days in the NICU were fully breastfed at discharge.

Procedure

Data were collected through review of patient medical records and by telephone interviews with mothers who had given their consent to participate after having received written information about the study and the contents of the interview. The interviews were conducted by the first author when the infants had reached the age of 3 months and lasted between 15 and 45 minutes. The following questions were posed during the interview:

(1) What advice can you give me as a nurse on how we can facilitate the initiation of breastfeeding in the NICU?

(2) What advice would you like to give another mother in the same situation as you were, trying to start breastfeeding in the NICU?

The answers were written down verbatim during the interview or as notes that were transcribed immediately thereafter. In order to secure its accuracy, the answer was repeated by the author, and the mother was asked whether it had been recorded correctly. Data collection and classification of contents occurred simultaneously and were made by the first author. The answers were divided according to themes so that the contents would not overlap, and were then brought together in categories. (For example, under the category 'Advice on breastfeeding' some of the themes were: Give advice as early as possible. Have a supportive attitude.) When more than one mother gave exactly the same comment or advice, this was scored as an additional observation of the theme/category in question. When the same person gave several comments concerning one category, these comments were recorded as separate themes and counted separately.

Classification

The classification of the answers on the basis of the adaptation theory was made independently by the first author and two other registered nurses, research assistants, in the NICU, who were not previously familiar with the theory. The material classified was the transcribed answers structured under themes and categories. The nurses were given a manual for classification containing a short description of the theory, and the adaptation modes with subheadings (see Table 8.1). They were asked to classify every theme if possible, otherwise the category, according to the adaptation mode concerned and respective subheading of the mode. They were also asked to consider whether the comments and advice were related to persons other than the mother and infant, and, if so, to classify these themes accordingly.

The classifications were compared in five different ways to test interrater reliability.

(1) Classification of every *th*eme according to the four adaptation modes with *s*ub-*h*eading (see Table 8.1) for *a*ll persons concerned – mother, infant, father, siblings and staff; TH-SH-A.
(2) Classification of every *th*eme according to the adaptation *m*odes (not divided into subheadings) for *a*ll persons concerned; TH-M-A.
(3) Classification of the *ca*tegories according to the adaptation modes with *s*ubheadings for *a*ll persons concerned; CAT-SH-A.
(4) Classification of every *th*eme according to the adaptation modes with *s*ubheadings for answers concerning only the *mo*ther; TH-SH-MO.
(5) Classification of the *ca*tegories according to the adaptation *m*odes (not

divided into subheadings) for answers concerning only the *mo*ther; CAT-M-MO.

The classification of all themes concerning mothers was compared to study the distribution on modes of themes on which at least two persons agreed about the classification. The themes and categories on which the first author and research assistants reached agreement (agreement by at least two persons) in their classification were then compiled to interpret the situation of the mother, the infant, the father and siblings and nurses according to the adaptation theory.

Results

Advice from mothers to NICU nurses on the facilitation of breastfeeding

The categories were ranked according to the total number of comments and advice, with advice for mothers delivered by a Caesarian section and for those delivered by vaginal delivery presented separately (Table 8.2). As several mothers gave more than one comment and piece of advice concerning the same category, the rank order should not be regarded as absolute, but rather as an indication of what mothers found important.

The majority of the comments and advice concerned the physical and the psychosocial environment in the NICU. The main advice concerned the need for privacy, to be able to sit and hold their baby, get acquainted with him and breastfeed without being looked at, and to dare to express feelings of joy and sadness. (For the sake of convenience infants will be called him.) Mothers felt uncomfortable in the technical and hectic environment with other sick infants, nurses, other parents and equipment. They found the unit stressful, hot and cramped. They thought that advice on breastfeeding should be given as a routine to all mothers as soon as possible, and that the mother – not nurses – should feed the baby. Feeding by bottle or gavage tube should be done only when absolutely necessary and the reason should be explained to the mother. Among mothers delivered by Caesarian section, the distance between the NICU and post-operative ward and the maternity wards caused the most problems, as they were forced to wait to see their baby and experienced trouble in getting assistance with transportation.

Advice to other mothers on the initiation of breastfeeding when the baby is in the NICU

The majority of advice (Table 8.3) focused on being calm and persistent and not giving up even if the infant is difficult to breastfeed or the mother is not allowed to breastfeed in the beginning. It is important to have physical contact with the infant and to start to breastfeed frequently as soon as

Table 8.2 Mothers' advice to NICU staff on the facilitation of breastfeeding: total number of comments/ advice from mothers delivered vaginally ($n = 79$) and those delivered by Caesarean section ($n = 99$)

Content of comments and advice	Total		Vaginal		Caesarean	
	Rank	No.	Rank	No.	Rank	No.
Physical environment in the NICU	1	178	1	119	2	59
Advice on breastfeeding	2	127	2	83	4	44
The distance between the NICU and the maternity unit/unit of gynaecological surgery	3	80	8	18	1	62
Feeding routines in the NICU	4	79	3	65	13	14
Organization of work: responsibility	5	62	4	43	9	19
Waiting in the post-operative ward	6	56	0	0	3	56
Behaviour towards parents: to be seen	7	51	5	32	11	19
Being a patient in a maternity ward	8	48	6	24	7	24
Information about the baby	9	43	9	16	5	27
The first visit to the NICU	10	39	19	15	6	24
Taking care of one's baby	11	29	7	21	14	8
Feelings of unreality, lack of maternal feelings, sadness	12	28	15	5	8	23
Discharge	13	27	12	10	12	17
Information when the baby was discharged from the NICU	14	22	15	3	10	19
Comments on breastfeeding in general	15	20	11	15	17	5
Behaviour towards the baby	16	11	14	6	18	5
Information before the delivery	17	10	13	7	19	3
The delivery/Caesarian section	18	8	17	1	15	7
Special problems in the NICU for mothers after Caesarean section	19	5	0	0	16	5

Table 8.3 Mothers' advice to other mothers on the initiation of breastfeeding when the baby is in the NICU, totally and for mothers delivered vaginally and by Caesarean section

Content of comments and advice	Total	Vaginal	Caesarean
Take it easy, do not give up	64	45	19
Contact with the baby	52	26	26
Breastfeed as soon and as often as possible	30	21	9
Ask the staff for advice and help	23	18	5
Take care of and feed your baby yourself	18	14	4
Sit in private	14	10	4
Use a breastpump to express your milk	14	9	5
Get help with transportation and decide the duration of your visit in the NICU	7	0	7
Feed your baby on demand, not fixed schedule	6	5	1

possible, and not to hesitate to ask nurses for advice. The mothers are told not to allow nurses to 'take over' the care and feeding of their infants.

Analysis according to Roy's adaptation theory

Interrater reliability

The classifications of themes according to the theory made by the first author and two research assistants were compared in five different ways (see earlier section on Procedure) and the number of themes/categories on which agreement was reached by three and by two persons was calculated (Table 8.4). The classification of every theme according to the subheadings of the adaptation theory for all persons concerned showed the lowest figure (74.3%) for agreement by at least two persons. Restriction of the classification of themes for all persons concerned to the modes without subheadings showed a slightly higher agreement, and a further restriction to categories and modes for all persons concerned showed an even higher figure. The highest agreement, however, was attained when the classification was limited to mothers: 90.5% for classification of themes according to subheadings, and 92.5% for categories according to modes. Thus, categories instead of themes showed higher consistency, as did a restriction of the classification to deal exclusively with themes concerning mothers.

An analysis of the distribution of modes in the classification of themes concerning mothers, on which at least two persons agreed about the classification, showed that only 31% of the themes were assigned to one mode (Table 8.5). There was considerable overlap of modes: 35.7% of the themes were assigned to two modes, 21% to three modes, and 8.3% to all four modes. In the 58 combinations of 2–4 modes, role functions occurred in 43 (74.1%), interdependence in 36 (62.1%), physiological needs in 32 (55.2%)

Table 8.4   Interrater agreement in the classification of advice from mothers in themes/categories according to the adaptation theory (n = number of themes/categories classified in each type of comparison)

Type of comparison*	Any combination						Total
	of three persons		of two persons		of at least two persons		
	n	%	n	%	n	%	n
TH-SH-A	110	35.7	119	38.6	229	74.3	308
TH-M-A	112	40.6	99	35.8	211	76.4	272
CAT-SH-A	91	61.9	31	21.1	122	83.0	147
TH-SH-MO	61	64.2	25	26.3	86	90.5	95
CAT-M-MO	25	62.5	12	30.0	37	92.5	40

*See classification section in text.

Table 8.5 Distribution and combinations of modes in the classification of themes concerning mothers (agreement by at least two persons)

One mode		Two modes		Three modes		Four modes		
Mode	*n*	Modes	*n*	Modes	*n*	Modes	*n*	Total
P	9	RS	7	RSI	10	PRSI	7	
R	7	IR	7	PRS	5			
I	7	PS	5	PSI	4			
S	3	PR	5	PRI	2			
		PI	4					
		SI	2					
	26 (31%)		30 (35.7%)		21 (25%)		7 (8.3%)	84 (100%)

P = Physiological needs, R = role functions, S = self-concept, I = interdependence, *n* = number of themes.

and self-concept in 30 (51.7%). Classifications showed all possible combinations of modes. The overlap was not limited to the three psychosocial modes, but was also frequent for physiological needs.

Contents of mothers' advice according to the adaptation theory

The main advice, on which at least two persons reached agreement in classification, was structured according to the adaptation theory as follows.

Mothers' physiological needs

Fluids/nutrition
Mothers experience difficulty in keeping times for meals, and may like something to drink in the NICU.

Protection
Pain implies the need for analgesics and assistance with transportation, and poses an obstacle to frequent visits to the unit, thus causing delays in meeting the infant and initiating breastfeeding. Mothers may need help to take care of their infant, to carry it and position the infant while nursing, comfortable chairs and a place to lie down. Breast soreness is prevented by correct positioning of the infant when nursing, and by regular expression of milk by breast pump when frequent visits are impossible.

Exercise and rest
The distance between the infants' and mothers' wards makes it difficult to find adequate time for rest, and the lack of privacy in the NICU makes it impossible to rest there. Mothers may feel forced to abstain from rest in order to take care of their infant.

All the senses
A stressful, technical environment affects the senses negatively.

Endocrine functions
Pain and discomfort, lack of rest, and stress because of the infant's care in the NICU affect hormones governing milk production and let-down reflex. Early physical contact with the infant, in private, is important for this process, as is adequate advice on the initiation of breastfeeding.

Mothers' role functions

Maternal role
To enter this new role, mothers need to examine their infant, participate actively in taking care of his needs, be informed about the infant's condition and care. Breastfeeding is an important expression of the maternal role, requiring extended physical contact in privacy, the acknowledgement by others of this role, knowledge of body functions and on the initiation of breastfeeding, and information on parents' role in the NICU. Feelings of unreality about the infant's birth, separation, delayed first contact, embarrassment in front of others, nurse behaviours and hospital routines are obstacles to this role.

Role as patient in the maternity ward
As mothers of patients spend most of their time in the NICU, they may miss information, feel that they do not fit into the pattern and find it difficult to share room with rooming-in mothers. They may adopt a passive patient role, not daring to ask questions and make demands, such as assistance with transportation to the NICU. After a Caesarean section, mothers may feel that they are denied a justified patient role and be expected to act as any other mother.

Role as parent of a patient
Systematic information should be given as soon as possible in the maternity ward and in the NICU on ward routines, the role of parents, and rules for visiting. Mothers may feel unprepared for the transition from this role to that of an ordinary parent when the baby is discharged.

Mothers' self-concept

Physical self
Mothers may need to talk about a difficult delivery or unplanned section to regain confidence in their body. Routines for feeding the infant with bottle or

gavage tube instead of encouraging breastfeeding, and omission of information about breastfeeding physiology and milk expression, may conserve
incorrect concepts of bodily functions.

Personal self

Self-consistency

Self-consistency is maintained when mothers are respected in their role, feel
welcome to the unit, are given appropriate attention, are expected to feed
their infant, preferably on demand, and realize that the infant will only spend
a very brief period of his life in hospital. It is supported by assistance with
transportation and encouragement of physical contact in private, and
hindered by lack of information, need for post-operative care, feelings of
unreality, and breastfeeding problems. If possible, mothers should be
informed in advance that their infant will need care in the NICU.

Self-ideal

Self-ideal is attained when mothers feel capable of meeting their infants'
needs, and feel competent when comparing themselves to other mothers and
staff. Obstacles are separation from the infant because of pain, fatigue and
problems with transportation, embarrassment in front of others, unrealistic
demands (by themselves or others on frequent visiting and on successful
breastfeeding), lack of information or assistance, hospital feeding routines,
hesitation to ask for information and advice, and the perception that nurses
take over their role.

Moral–ethical self

Moral–ethical self concerns feelings of guilt: about delayed first contact with
the infant, for missing information and routines in the maternity ward. It also
concerns the right of parents to question medical procedures and hospital
routines. Some mothers may consider it unethical to breastfeed in front of
others.

Mothers' interdependence

Mothers depend on nurses for their own and the infant's physiological needs,
for physical contact with the infant, for permission to take care of the infant,
for initiation of breastfeeding, and for confidence in view of discharge.
Transition towards independence is facilitated when mothers feel secure
when absent from the infant, and are allowed to take their infant's care at an
individual pace. Obstacles are lack of routines for information and lack of
sensitivity to mothers' wishes, when nurses take over the maternal role in

decision-making and care and make mothers feel that they 'disturb' them by asking questions.

Infants' physiological needs

Fluid and electrolyte balance, nutrition
The administration of nutrients should be adapted in a flexible way to medical needs and individual cues. The prescription of big volumes by bottle or gavage tube, in spite of being necessary, may have a negative influence on infants' ability to suck their mothers' breast, cause spitting up and vomiting, and delay the initiation of breastfeeding. The goal should be on-demand feeding.

Protection
Infants should not be allowed to lie crying for a long time unconsoled, and feeding sessions should not be interrupted for drawing of blood samples.

Exercise and rest
Routines should be adjusted to infants' sleep–wake rhythm and cues of hunger.

The senses
Infants need close physical contact with their parents, preferably skin-to-skin.

Endocrine functions
Physical contact with the parents in a quiet environment, in private, and a caring attitude among nurses reduce stress.

Infants' role and self-concept

Allowing infants to start sucking their mothers' breast, to show their competence, is a way of letting them experience who they are and of respecting their role as a child.

Infants' interdependence

Infants depend on nurses for the transition to feeding according to their individual cues, on demand.

Fathers' physiological needs

Immediate information about the infants' condition reduces anxiety and stress.

Fathers' role functions

In connection with Caesarian sections, fathers serve an important function by being present and by informing the mother afterwards of what has happened and of the condition and care of the infant. To do so they need information, attention and encouragement to take an active part in the infant's care.

Fathers' interdependence

Independence in the paternal role is supported by information about rules for visiting, instruction on the infant's care and availability for assistance, and by nurse behaviour that inspires father's trust that the infant is in good hands. Diffuse information about the infant's condition and waiting for discharge from the NICU may cause disagreement between fathers and nurses.

Nurses' role functions

There should be a system for the assignment of responsibility for each patient in the NICU and in the maternity ward. Nurses should give required health care, constantly adjust routines to meet changing needs, have routines for information, give priority to breastfeeding, and provide a quiet environment with privacy. For a clear demarcation between roles, nurses should encourage the maternal role by giving adequate instruction about infant care and feeding, and try to prevent feeding of estrangement in the maternity ward. They should facilitate normal parent/infant interaction by arranging visits according to parents' wishes, involving mothers in care planning and by supporting them in taking over responsibility.

Discussion

The purpose of this study was to classify, structure and interpret advice from patients' mothers on the initiation of breastfeeding in accordance with Roy's theory and to test interrater reliability in the classification. Mothers' advice to nurses concerned mainly the NICU environment, advice on breastfeeding and need of physical contact. It frequently touched upon nurse behaviours related to mothers' perceived difficulties in entering the maternal role. Their advice to other mothers, with a focus on persistence and confidence in one's ability to breastfeed, and early physical contact, also stressed the right of mothers to take care of and feed their infants.

The classification of the data by the first author and two nurses according to Roy's theory showed a high degree of agreement, but also considerable overlap of the four adaptation modes, displaying all possible combinations of two, three or four modes in the classification of themes. This classification was then used to operationalize the theory in a description of the situation of mothers, infants, fathers and nurses.

Mothers' advice appeared to give a somewhat different priority to main factors influencing the initiation of breastfeeding, compared to what is reported in current literature. As in the literature, mothers stressed the importance of early extensive physical contact and the need of structured information. In addition, they gave extensive advice on specific components in the NICU environment they perceived as obstacles. The essence of this advice concerned reactions to lack of privacy and perceived lack of respect for the maternal (and paternal) roles among nurses. A number of hospital routines and nurse behaviours, such as organization of transportation, rigid feeding schedules, and lack of systematic advice on breastfeeding, were interpreted as indifference to the parental role and to the importance of breastfeeding for both mother and infant. This confirms the need of an institutional philosophy, which is transmitted to patients in nurse actions and attitudes (Cohen, 1987).

Mothers considered it a major nurse role function to encourage parents to enter their new role by facilitating undisturbed parent/infant contact and active parent participation in the infant's care and feeding. Nurses should take it for granted that breastfeeding on demand is the obvious main goal of the care plan, unless parents explicitly express a different opinion. Steps to change the physical environment should be taken to increase privacy in every possible way for parents, in order to allow expression of emotions and prevent embarrassment. From mothers' description of events and nurse behaviours, it appears crucial that nurses are fully aware of the impact of their behaviour and nursing routines on patients and parents, and that nurses have a consensus on attitudes, which is observable in routines for care and information. One way of sharing such a consensus is the application of a nursing theory.

Application of theory

In order to evaluate the application of a nursing theory to a certain clinical setting, instruments have to be tested for their efficacy. In order for a theory to be practicable as the ideological foundation for the nursing process it must have such a clear structure that nurses can easily (a) be instructed to understand and use it, and (b) be able to do so in a uniform way. The present study was undertaken to test the agreement in nurses' classification of mothers' advice and comments after having received instructions about the theory in a format that may be realistic to use for instruction purposes in a clinical setting. In a research setting, interrater reliability is normally tested by comparing the scores of two persons who have received extensive training in the procedure concerned. This is not feasible in a clinal setting.

To add strength to the test undertaken in this study, three persons, instead of just two, classified data which were then analysed for agreement. The choice of interview responses instead of patient/parent situations in a daily clinical working situation for the classification provided several advantages: the first author and research assistants could classify the same data, and there was a sufficient amount of data to allow an extensive analysis of the classification.

The magnitude of agreement reached in this study can be compared to studies on reliability concerning psychiatric diagnoses, where agreements between two of five experienced psychiatrists ranged between 48% and 72%, and kappa coefficients between 0.54 and 0.80 (Eysenck *et al.*, 1983). Although there was a considerable difference between the magnitude of agreement between two and three persons in the present study, the overall degree of agreement by at least two persons ranged between 74% and 92%, which is much higher than in the studies quoted above. This also indicates that Roy's theory is sufficiently easy to understand and apply, even after a brief introduction.

The main problem encountered in the classification of data and in the evaluation of the classification was a lack of clarity in the distinction between modes. For example, the comparison of classifications of themes supports the critique that the psychosocial modes (role functions, self-concept and inter-dependence) cannot be distinguished from each other clearly enough to allow consistent classification. This overlap of modes was evident not only for the psychosocial modes; the physiological mode also occurred more frequently in combinations with other modes than alone. The research assistants remarked that the close connection between the psychosocial adaptation modes made it possible only occasionally to classify a theme as concerning merely one mode or one subheading. They reported that they frequently selected a certain mode or subheading only because it seemed more pertinent to the theme, not because the others did not apply. The subheadings under self-concept, for example, were given widely different classifications.

The choice made often seemed to depend on the time aspect: if the mother's situation was looked upon as here and now, the theme was classified as 'ideal self', but if the situation was looked upon as part of a process over time, it was classified as 'self-consistency'. However, it is the authors' opinion that the fact that one theme could concern several modes and sub-headings does not necessarily have to be interpreted as a shortcoming of the theory, but rather as a confirmation of the complexity of nursing situations with several simultaneous overlapping patient needs. It may even illustrate the inappropriateness of limiting the assessment in the nursing process to lists of patient needs according to simplistic protocols. On the other hand, this also corroborates the opinion that tests of so called grand theories are problematic, because the abstract theoretical constructs do not lend themselves easily to empirical application (Acton *et al.* 1991).

A further reason for incongruence classification was that the first author and research assistants related their classifications of some of the themes/categories to different persons. This appears to be the main reason why agreement was only reached for few of the classifications regarding fathers and especially siblings, which were therefore excluded from the structured interpretation. Role functions were not specified by either author or research assistants as primary, secondary or tertiary, as such a specification requires an assessment of the individual's total situation, about which data were not available in this study.

Fruitfulness of theory

In the debate on nursing theories, critique has been raised that nursing theories are rarely tested, remaining primarily on a descriptive level. According to another view, the purpose of nursing theories is to describe phenomena in order to reach understanding, and make explanations and predictions. A theory will then not necessarily have to be tested as such (Rooke, 1990). Instead, the value of the practical application of a theory should be judged according to its fruitfulness: whether new insight and suggestions are generated in the process. A combination of these two views on the usefulness of nursing theories could be that theories should be tested in research that evaluates how well the explanations that evolve from a theory lead to a clearer and more useful depiction of reality.

If the interpretation and structuring of mothers' advice according to Roy's theory is judged from the point of fruitfulness, it:

(1) Provided an empirical background for operationalization of the theory in the NICU setting.
(2) Served to identify a large number of stress factors as well as several suggestions on what may be regarded as positive stimuli, factors that can be used for facilitating the parental role and normalizing infants' experience in the NICU.
(3) Provided a framework for the clarification of a nurse role, which is in agreement with parents' concept of a division of role functions that supports the parental roles.
(4) Assisted in a deeper understanding of the complex interaction between infant/parents and numerous components in the NICU environment.

Based on the criterion of fruitfulness, the application of adaptation theory can be considered one way of contributing to quality nursing care.

The extensive overlap of modes in the classification, however, gives reason to doubt the appropriateness of applying the theory as such to the daily assessment of patient needs according to the nursing process. For this purpose, the theory should be made operational by applying it as a framework for designing concrete assessment tools, adapted to particular nursing settings. Such tools can then be tested for their possible contribution to better outcomes. The test should naturally include patients' own evaluation of nursing routines and nurse behaviour.

Conclusion

In spite of problems in distinctions between modes, the adaptation theory has the capacity for practical application in an NICU and for enhancing quality nursing, in its function as a theoretical framework for description, explanation and understanding the situation of mothers, infants, fathers and siblings. The present study demonstrated that this is true under the condition that one important addition is made to its basic structure: the incorporation of the interactive aspect of the attitudes, role functions and behaviour of nurses, and how these are perceived by patients and their families.

With this revision, it can be used as an instrument for structuring nursing activities in an NICU in a way that prevents role conflicts between nurses and parents and that leaves parents confident that their infant is in good care in their absence. This is in line with the view of a reciprocal relationship between theory and practice, meaning that conceptual models are not to be regarded as ideologies that cannot be changed. On the contrary, their credibility should be tested in the real world of clinical practice and revised accordingly (Fawcett, 1992). The experience of interpreting the data according to the theory was described by one research assistant as suddenly facing a new image of activities in the NICU as a continuous game materialized in role conflicts between nurses and parents. Such an insight can serve as a foundation for shaping a professional role that is more finely attuned to the expectations and convictions of patients and their families.

The impact of the theory on nurses' concept of their professional role functions related to patients and their relatives, based on attitudes, conscious or unconscious, and displayed in behaviours, needs to be tested further in order to establish the value of its practical application.

Acknowledgements

This study was supported by a grant from the Gillbergska Foundation, Uppsala. The authors wish to express grateful thanks to the research assistants, Anne-Maj Ling, RN and Lena Svensson, RN, Neonatal Intensive Care

Unit 95F, University Hospital, Uppsala, for their participation in the classification and helpful comments.

References

Acton, G.J., Irvin, B.L., Hopkins, B.A. (1991) Theory-testing research: building the science. *Advances in Nursing Science*, **1**, 52–61.

Cohen, S.P. (1987) High tech – soft touch: breastfeeding issues. *Clinics in Perinatology*, **14**(1), 187–96.

Eysenck, H.J., Wakefield, J.A. & Friedman, A.F. (1983) Diagnosis and clinical assessment: the DSM-III. *Annual Review of Psychology*, **34**, 167–93.

Fawcett, J. (1992) Conceptual models and nursing practice: the reciprocal relationship. *Journal of Advanced Nursing*, **17** 224–8.

Fawcett, J. & Tulman, L. (1990) Building a programme of research from the Roy Adaptation Model of Nursing. *Journal of Advanced Nursing*, **15**, 720–25.

Galligan, A.C. (1979) Using Roy's concept of adaptation to care for young children. *American Journal of Maternal Child Nursing*, Jan/Feb, 24–8.

Hamner, J.B. (1989) Applying the Roy adaptation model to the CCU. *Critical Care Nurse*, **9**(3), 51–61.

Jackson, D.A. (1990) Roy in the postanesthesia care unit. *Journal of Post Anesthesia Nursing*, **5**(3), 143–8.

Miles, M.S. & Carter, M.C. (1983) Assessing parental stress in intensive care units. *American Journal of Maternal Child Nursing*, **8**, Sep/Oct, 354–9.

Munn, V.A. & Tichy, A.M. (1987) Nurses' perceptions of stressors in pediatric intensive care. *Journal of Pediatric Nursing*, **2**(6), 405–11.

Norberg, A. & Wickstrom, E. (1990) The perception of Swedish nurses and nurse teachers of the integration of theory with nursing practice. An explorative qualitative study. *Nurse Education Today*, **10**(1), 38–43.

Norris, S., Campbell, L.A. & Brenkert, S. (1982) Nursing procedures and alterations in transcutaneous oxygen tension in premature infants. *Nursing Research*, **31**(6), 330–36.

Rooke, L. (1990) Nursing and theoretical structures of nursing: a didactic attempt to develop the practice of nursing. Doctoral thesis, University of Lund. *Studia Psychologica et Pedagogica, series altera XCVI*. Almquist & Wiksell International, Stockholm.

Roy, C. (1980) The Roy adaptation model. In *Conceptual Models for Nursing Practice*, 2nd edn (eds J.P. Riehl & C. Roy) pp. 179–88. Appleton–Century–Crofts, New York.

Roy, C. & Roberts, S.L. (1981) *Theory Construction in Nursing. An Adaptation Model*. Englewood Cliffs, Prentice-Hall, New Jersey.

Silva, C.S. (1986) Research testing nursing theory: state of the art. *Advances in Nursing Science*, **9** 1–11.

Silva, M.C., Sorrel, J.M. (1992) Testing of nursing theory: critique and philosophical expansion. *Advances in Nursing Science*, **4** 12–23.

Wagner, P. (1976) Testing the Adaptation Model in practice. *Nursing Outlook*, **24**(11), 682–5.

Chapter 9
Mitral valve prolapse and its effects: a programme of inquiry within Orem's Self-Care Deficit Theory of Nursing

SHARON WILLIAMS UTZ, *PhD, RN*

Associate Professor, School of Nursing, University of Virginia

and MARY CAROL RAMOS, *PhD, RN*

Quality Management Co-ordinator, Division of Health Care Evaluation, University of Virginia Hospital, Charlottesville, Virginia, USA

The optimum growth and scientific progress of nursing knowledge during the next century will depend upon the development and execution of focused programmes of clinical and theoretical research. The planning and design of such programmes must originate with the clear definition of nursing research questions. Nesting such questions within established theoretical frameworks provides a nursing context, lends precise language and suggests relevant variables for study. The development of a sequence of related studies exploring and describing the self-care needs of people with symptomatic mitral valve prolapse illustrates one such systematic research programme. Orem's Self-Care Deficit Theory of Nursing was used as a theoretical framework for four completed studies which describe one population's need for nursing assistance. The evolving nature of the research programme and plans for future research are discussed.

Introduction

As the health care system expands and becomes more complex, the role of nursing and the scope of nursing knowledge evolve. It has been established that clinical nursing inquiry will be integral to the development of new health care roles and the appreciation of new nursing knowledge. The optimum growth and diversification of such knowledge during the next century will be maximized by the development of focused research programmes by nurse scholars. While single studies contribute to nursing knowledge, a series of projects, each predicated upon previous conclusions, is a powerful tool for the advancement of the discipline.

Several nurse authors have encouraged such programmes of nursing research (Chance & Hinshaw, 1980; Schlodtfeldt, 1986; Stevenson, 1988; Williams, 1989). Chance & Hinshaw (1980) described the importance of a unified, co-ordinated research effort within any complex organization. Stevenson (1988) also emphasized the importance of systematic planning and discussed various strategies to maximize the sharing of research expertise, including mentor roles for seasoned researchers and the use of collaborative group projects. She asserted that developing such programmes of inquiry is truly the 'challenge for academic nursing' in the next few decades. Williams (1989) discussed the difficulties of developing this important approach for new nurse academicians. The scarcity of mentors and heavy clinical teaching responsibilities are barriers to comprehensive, systematic research planning.

There is also a paucity of descriptions concerning research programmes within the nursing literature. A few examples describe a unified, co-ordinated approach to the answering of related nursing research questions (Cole & Slocumb, 1990; Fawcett & Tulman, 1990; Tomlinson *et al.*, 1986). Such papers help beginning nurse scholars better understand research programmes and identify some strategies for programme implementation. However, if research programmes are to be used confidently and consistently, more detailed exemplars are needed in the literature.

Most nursing research programmes begin with a clinical question, problem or incident. Well-explicated, nursing-based research questions are the origin of the most successful programmes. As Schlodtfeldt (1986) astutely noted, the discipline of nursing cannot depend upon scientists in other health disciplines who cannot frame research questions in the same way as do nurse scientists. To assure further disciplinary grounding, nursing questions can be nested within an extant nursing theory framework. A framework that is clearly nursing based – as opposed to frameworks drawn from psychology, physiology or other human sciences – can enhance a systematic programme by supplying a set of assumptions, precise terminology and, indeed, some of the variables for a series of studies.

This chapter describes an example of a programme of research, a programme designed to explore and define the nursing needs of a population of people with symptomatic mitral valve prolapse. Orem's Theory of Self-Care Deficit Nursing was utilized as a framework.

The clinical problem

The health deviation known as mitral valve prolapse (MVP) is one that has been described in the medical literature as an innocuous structural variant or a 'benign syndrome' (Devereux, 1989; Levy & Savage, 1987; MacMahon *et al.*, 1987). Mitral valve prolapse is an alteration in the structure and function of the cardiac mitral valve; it occurs when there is 'posterior and superior systolic displacement of the mitral leaflets in relation to the mitral annulus, due to structural enlargement or abnormal distensibility of the mitral valve' (Perloff & Child, 1987). Approximately 4%–5% of American adults, or seven million people, have been diagnosed with MVP (Devereux, 1989; Levy & Savage, 1987). It is the general consensus of physicians that MVP is not a 'disease', although it is frequently diagnosed and the majority of those diagnosed report troublesome symptoms associated with the finding (MacMahon *et al.*, 1987).

Health risks

Symptoms and health risks vary enormously among people with MVP (MacMahon *et al.*, 1987); at least two diagnostic subgroups exist (Marks *et al.*, 1989). One small group (less than 1%) is at risk for serious complications such as embolism, endocarditis or sudden death. These patients require vigilant, episodic medical evaluation and nursing care centring on teaching and health promotion within the limitations of the physical deviation (Grass & Utz, 1986).

The vast majority (99 + %) of people diagnosed with MVP, however, have the 'non-classic' form, a condition which reportedly does not significantly alter mortality (Levy & Savage, 1987; MacMahon *et al.*, 1987; Perloff & Child, 1987). However, all have a five-fold risk of infective endocarditis and an estimated 50%–75% exhibit noticeable symptoms (Marks *et al.*, 1989).

MVP patients commonly seek medical assistance for troubling symptoms such as chest pain, palpitations, shortness of breath, syncope and severe fatigue (Grass & Utz, 1986). Physicians commonly 'reassure' their patients that MVP is a benign finding (Anderson, 1990), but patients report that such reassurance does not necessarily help in symptom management. Studies by the present authors and others have shown that symptoms often remain unchanged or, perhaps, are exacerbated by feelings of fear, frustration and isolation (Anderson, 1990; MacMahon *et al.*, 1987; Utz *et al.*, 1990).

Although people with symptomatic MVP may not find a medical cure, they may be greatly assisted through nursing care. Because nursing care focuses on the person within a social, psychological and biological context, nurses are prepared to compile an integrated, holistic data set. Using these assessments, nurses can facilitate lifestyle changes which may alter symptoms, decrease health risks and enhance psychological comfort (Allan & Hall, 1988). However, the ability to provide nursing for people with MVP is severely limited by a lack of direct access to nurses and by the paucity of published empirical nursing knowledge to guide nursing practice.

Anecdotal information

Until recent years, the nursing literature was limited to anecdotal information, such as Simonetti's (1980) descriptions of her own severe chest pain associated with MVP. Cash & Grissett (1985) later provided a more comprehensive description of the variety of symptoms associated with MVP, emphasizing what they described as 'life devastating' experiences with the condition.

The present researchers and colleagues have enlarged the literature by reviewing medical literature on MVP (Grass & Utz, 1986) and by describing clinical observations organized according to a theoretical framework, Orem's Theory of Self-Care Deficit Nursing (Utz & Grass, 1987). The series of studies described in this chapter was designed to address multiple unanswered nursing questions and deficiencies in nursing knowledge.

Orem's Theory as a research framework

The nursing model chosen as an orienting framework for these studies was Orem's Self-Care Deficit Theory of Nursing (Orem, 1991). As indicated in Fig. 9.1, the focus of nursing is upon a person's need for self-care (A). Based on a careful assessment of a person's health-care needs (therapeutic self-care demands, B) and his or her resources for meeting those self-care demands (self-care agency, C), the nurse can evaluate any deficiencies that exist (self-care deficit, D). In this process, the nurse must be aware of the client's mental abilities (including decision-making skill) and perceptions of his or her own health state, including health-related knowledge and goals.

Nursing assessment also includes an evaluation of the client's physical and emotional ability to value and pursue optimum health. To the best of his or her capabilities within the relationship and the context of conditioning factors such as gender and cultural background, the nurse strives to understand the patient's perspective. For example, nurses understand that a medical diagnosis (in this case, of MVP) may carry a unique meaning for the individual; nursing assistance is designed to be consonant with that meaning. Given this assessment, the practitioner can plan care to augment the patient's capabilities and provide necessary assistance in self-care (nursing agency E).

Orem's framework provides a nursing-based focus and systematic guidelines for examining the balance between patients' needs, capabilities and limitations in exercising self-care actions to enhance personal health. Through the use of an educative-supportive nursing system (Orem, 1991), skilled nursing can assist a client to acquire knowledge, skills and a sense of self-efficacy with which to manage his or her own health. Orem's framework

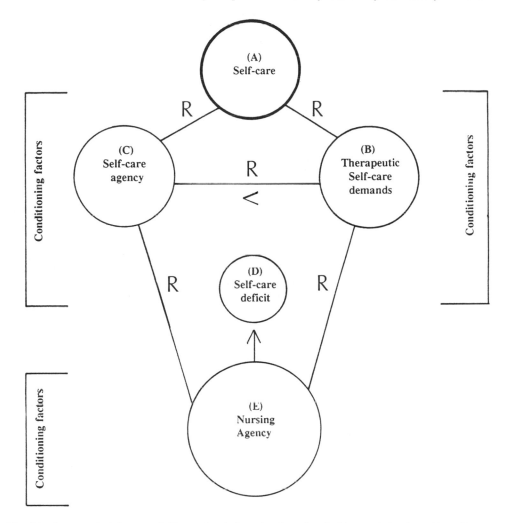

Fig. 9.1 A conceptual framework for nursing (adapted and reprinted with permission from Orem D. (1991) *Nursing: Concepts of Practice* 4th edn. Mosby Year Books, St Louis). R = relationships; R < R = current or projected deficit relationship.

thus provides a method for identifying and attending to each patient's unique needs and capabilities.

Orem's model of nursing practice therefore addresses several characteristics of MVP as a nursing problem. First, Orem's model requires that the client's perspective is integral to assessing needs and planning nursing assistance. Since MVP is not considered a 'legitimate disease' by most physicians, those diagnosed are often confused regarding the relative seriousness of their condition. The framework also incorporates an assessment of the patient's knowledge of his or her condition.

Often patients are not given detailed explanations of the physiological aspects of MVP. They have the dissonant experience of being told that the condition is benign when their symptoms certainly do not seem benign. This dissonance can easily be incorporated into Orem's model of assessment, planning and evaluation of care. Furthermore, Orem's framework is focused upon a person's capabilities and limitations for self-care. In planning and implementing ongoing health care, the nurse can use this knowledge to assist a person toward optimum self-care.

While the use of Orem's framework was intuitively attractive, actual assessment in this population was limited by a lack of research-based information concerning the impact of symptomatic MVP. The terminology and its applicability to planning the care of those with symptomatic MVP needed clarification and empirical validation. Therefore, a series of nursing studies was planned and implemented. The four described studies formed the essence of a programme of nursing research using Orem's model (Table 9.1). Each study, described briefly, contributed a unique facet to the evolving research programme.

Table 9.1 Specific components of Orem's theory studied.

Study	Components of SCDNT*

(1) Review:
124 medical records and
interviews: 20 symptomatic respondents
	Basic conditioning factors
	Health team perspective (medical)
	Self-care demands
	   Health deviation self-care requisites
	   Client perspective

(2) Interviews: Content analysis health concept	Perspective (client) Self-care demands
(3) Survey: 32 cardiovascular nurses in US	Health team perspective (nursing)

(4) Questionnaire:
Health State
  50 respondents
	Self-care demands
	   Health deviation self-care requisites
	   Client perspective

Planned studies	
(5) Revised questionnaire to national sample/ self-care agency scale	Self-care demands Self-care agency Self-care deficits

(6) Physiological study
  breathing patterns
  nursing prescription
	Methods of nursing assistance/effectiveness

*Self-Care Deficit Nursing Theory.

Study 1: self-care needs

Extant medical research and copious clinical nursing experience led researchers to the belief that people with symptomatic MVP had nursing care needs that could be addressed successfully through the use of Orem's framework. However, patients' self-care needs (therapeutic self-care demands) had not been defined and validated through clinical research. Thus, the research question driving this initial study was: What are the therapeutic self-care demands of people with symptomatic MVP?

A biphasic study was planned; interview data were ultimately desired, but medical record review was completed to allow for the identification of possible respondents, collection of demographic data, and an initial understanding of physicians' views of the condition. Permission for the study was sought from the Medical Centre Human Subjects Review Committee. Peer reviewers allowed review of medical records without reservation, but required physician notification and approval before patients were contacted for interviews in order to assure that patients were themselves aware of their MVP diagnosis.

Phase 1: Review of medical records

In Orem's framework, therapeutic self-care demands are determined through nursing assessment of health state, conditioning factors and self-care requisites (Fig. 9.1). Information concerning the medical component of such factors was sought from 124 patients' medical records containing a physician's diagnosis of MVP confirmed by two-dimensional echocardiography. Patient records were obtained from selected medical centre clinics and private physicians' offices in north-western Ohio, USA. Ages of these patients ranged from 18 to 69 ($\bar{x}$ = 34 years). The sample was 66% female, 85% white, 11% black and 1% each Asian and Hispanic.

Data obtained from the records included demographic information and general health status (basic conditioning factors), reported symptoms, voiced 'complaints' and medical diagnoses and prescribed treatments as recorded by physicians. While these data yielded only the medical perspective they were a valuable introduction to understanding one component of therapeutic self-care demands. It was noted, for example, that the most frequent medical treatments described for this group of patients were prescriptions for prophylactic antibiotics and beta-adrenergic antagonists ('beta blockers').

Data regarding therapeutic self-care demands were incomplete. Patients' capabilities or their willingness to adopt the prescribed medical regimens were not described. Only those aspects of MVP treatment considered noteworthy by one sample of physicians appeared in the records. Therefore, the usefulness of this information was severely limited within Orem's framework or any true nursing approach requiring biopsychosocial information (Allan & Hall, 1988). However, data describing the medical perspective were compiled and preliminarily analysed; demographic data and frequencies of patient concerns were noted. The next step was to add to the data base by compiling information concerning the clients' perspectives.

Phase 2: Interviews of people with symptomatic mitral valve prolapse

The second phase of the study focused explicitly upon obtaining the clients' perspective by selecting interview respondents from those whose records were reviewed. The exploratory, interactive approach was deemed an appropriate step toward the construction of an empirical instrument.

Sample

Participation was solicited from people whose medical records mentioned one or more 'typical symptoms'. Potential respondents were assured that the research team, nurse experts in the treatment of mitral valve prolapse, would be available to answer any questions they had about their condition, at the time of their interview. Twenty people agreed to participate. They ranged in age from 18 to 69 ($\bar{x}$ = 40 years); 60% was female and all were Caucasian.

Data collection and analysis

An exploratory interview protocol was chosen to maximize the richness of data concerning the experience with MVP (Spradley, 1979), including the context of diagnosis, perceived health effects and perceived life changes attributed to MVP. A semi-structured interview guide was developed to assure the acquisition of an appropriate data base. Items from the interview protocol were examined by three peer reviewers. Pilot interviews were conducted and instrument revision undertaken to increase clarity. Interviews began with open-ended questions about general experiences with the diagnosis of MVP and progressed to questions more specific to Orem's (1991) six categories of health deviation self-care requisites (Table 9.2).

All interviews were audiotaped, transcribed and read by the research team. Data were compiled and emic statements were extracted that expressed perceived meaning. Data bytes were then sorted into a preliminary *a priori* category system suggested by the theoretical framework. Those data that fitted into *a priori* categories of health deviation requisites were written on cards and sorted independently by the researchers and validated (93% agreement) through independent sortings.

Table 9.2 Interview questions based on health deviation self-care requisites (adapted from Orem 1985).

1. Seeking and securing appropriate medical assistance for health problem/converns:
   When do you seek health care for MVP?
   To whom do you go?
   How often do you seek care for this problem?
2. Being aware of and attending to effects and results of pathological conditions/states:
   How do you become aware of symptoms or problems related to MVP?
   What effects do these symptoms or problems have on you?
3. Effectively carrying out medically prescribed diagnostic, therapeutic or rehabilitation measures:
   What recommendations has your physician made about taking care of yourself in relation to MVP?
   Are you able to carry out the measures prescribed?
   If yes, what actions do you take? If not, why not?
4. Being aware of and attending to or regulating discomforting or deleterious effects of medical care measures:
   Have you noticed any problems or ill-effects from the prescribed meds/diet/exercise?
   If so, how do you deal with these?
   Do the above (medications/actions) help?
   Is the level of relief sufficient?
5. Modifying self-concept (and self-image) in accepting oneself as being in a particular state of health and in need of specific forms of health care:
   How has MVP affected the way you view yourself?
   Would you describe yourself any differently now than you did before you knew you had MVP?
6. Learning to live with effects of pathological conditions and effects of treatment measures in a lifestyle that promotes continued personal development
   What changes have you made in your daily life patterns or ways of taking care of yourself since you were told that you have MVP?

Findings

Data reflected expressed concerns in all six categories of health deviation self-care requisites (Table 9.2). Predominant concerns included perceived needs for:

(1) Acceptance by others (including health care personnel) of subjective discomfort.
(2) An understanding of the condition.
(3) Help with symptom management and lifestyle adjustment.

Nearly all of those interviewed asked for a clear explanation of the condition and how to interpret their symptoms. Common responses included, 'How do I know I'm not having a heart attack?' Additionally, they wanted to communicate successfully to health care personnel how dramatically the MVP symptoms had affected their lives.

Many felt dissatisfied with the care they had received and were looking for help. They verbalized a need for help with the prevention of complications which might further endanger their health.

Conclusions

Findings from this initial study were helpful in the identification of general pattern of help-seeking, perceived needs for assistance, levels of understanding concerning the condition, and comparative individual success with symptom management. Data suggested that the symptomatic subgroup of MVP patients is one for which nursing may have much to offer. The prevalence and consistency of this group's verbalized concerns and respondents' eagerness for information also supported the need for additional nursing research. It was recognized that the small, self-selected sample and geographical homogeneity of the preliminary study precluded generalizability. This led to the planning of a subsequent study (study 3), asking whether nurses in other areas of the country were consistently identifying similar needs.

Study 2: analysis of health perceptions and body image

While initial research questions about the self-care needs of people with symptomatic MVP were preliminarily answered in the first study, the data obtained through the interview process were of unexpected richness. Further analysis of client perspectives and therapeutic self-care demands was needed. The second study evolved because *a priori* categories did not encompass the total content of unanticipated, detailed verbalization concerning body image and perceptions of health (Utz *et al.*, 1990).

Since the first study had used Orem's categories of health-deviation self-care requisites to organize the interview guide, certain questions addressed topics of self-perception as related to the diagnosis of MVP (Table 9.2, category 5). These questions led to complex descriptions of respondents' views of their health and references to body images before and after diagnosis. The emergent research questions guiding study 2 were posed:

(1) What are this sample's most frequent perceptions of health?
(2) Do those diagnosed with MVP describe themselves in ways that reflect an altered body image associated with their diagnosis?

Data analysis

Earlier sortings of the data (study 1) had left a quantity of emic statements that could not be adequately categorized. These statements were preliminarily sorted into categories whose names seemed, at that point, to reflect meaning regarding health conceptions. From further reading in the nursing literature and from discussions between members of the research team, it was discovered that the data bytes could be grouped into three of the four classifications of health conceptions described by Smith (1981): (a) clinical, (b) role performance/functional, and (c) adaptational.

Smith's fourth category, eudemonistic perceptions, was applicable to statements made by two subjects. Body image descriptions were defined based on the literature, and were subsequently identified in 19 of the 20 transcripts, reflecting dominant concerns regarding body structure and function changes, and the meaning of particular sensory experiences associated with MVP.

Thus, the second study provided a detailed analysis of unanticipated issues regarding health conception and body image. These data provided valuable insight into the experiences of some people with symptomatic MVP, but also raised additional questions about whether this sample of 20 subjects was representative of common needs in this population. The researchers again noted that knowledge of the nursing perspective was needed to continue to expand understanding of clients' help-seeking patterns and to identify current nursing practice with this client population. Therefore, the next study was designed to collect data regarding nurses' experiences with patients with MVP as well as to address the external validity of results.

Study 3: a survey of cardiovascular nurses

The nurses' perspective about providing assistance to patients with MVP was sought through a survey sampling patients in differing practice settings across the United States. The research questions driving this study were:

(1) What health problems are most frequently observed by nurses caring for clients with MVP?
(2) What methods of nursing assistance are commonly utilized by these practitioners?

A prospectus of the study was presented to the Human Subjects Committee of Medical Centre. Since it was determined that return of the questionnaire would constitute consent to participate, the study was classified 'exempt'.

Sample

Nurses who had published in cardiovascular nursing journals, served on editorial boards and/or presented papers at cardiac nursing conferences were solicited as respondents through the mail. This circumscribed population was sampled in this initial study to increase the probability that respondents would be acquainted with MVP as a condition and with the related literature. A two-page questionnaire, consisting of checklists of symptoms and problems commonly seen in MVP and a list of typical nursing interventions, with space for additional comments, was mailed to 83 nurses; 34 usable surveys were returned (response rate of 42%). The resulting sample was predominantly female (93%), aged 32–45 ($\bar{x}$ = 37) and clinically experienced ($\bar{x}$ number of years in practice = 14). The five most frequent clinical symptoms reported by these nurses in patients with MVP were chest pain (53%), arrhythmias (53%), syncope (50%), anxiety (38%), shortness of breath (26%), migraines (20%) and numbness and/or tingling of extremities (12%).

Findings

Respondents reported that the methods of nursing assistance used for clients with MVP included teaching, supporting/guiding, and acting for or doing for patients (Table 9.3). These findings replicated those indicating that nurses tend to focus on providing information and recommending self-care actions, which may include recommending medications. In contrast, results from the medical records examined in study 1 indicated that physicians' primary recommendations were almost solely for prescription drugs.

Several nurse respondents asked questions indicating a lack of knowledge concerning MVP. Others expressed frustration with the fact that physicians 'spend time and money diagnosing the condition and then dismiss it as unimportant'. Nearly all respondents indicated difficulty with evaluation of nursing assistance owing to limited access to patients, the episodic nature of medical care and limited use of case management.

Table 9.3 Most frequently utilized nursing interventions reported by practitioners ($n = 32$)*.

(1) Teaching	(70%)
(2) Guiding/supporting:	(Total = 35%)
Counselling	(53%)
Recommending relaxation	(38%)
Recommending exercise	(35%)
Recommending diet change	(27%)
Recommended biofeedback	(12%)
(3) Acting for/doing for:	
recommending medications	(41%)

*Categories based on Orem (1985).

Conclusions

The findings of this survey, while limited by a small sample size and low response rate, can nonetheless be seen as supporting findings from the previous studies: there is a vulnerable subgroup of those with symptomatic MVP for whom nursing approaches could be beneficial. Additionally, experienced clinicians verbalized frustration with their inability to assess and evaluate the relative benefits of nursing assistance. As previously noted by this research team, a need for further empirical work exists.

Thus, the three completed studies provided a variety of data to begin filling knowledge gaps concerning the needs of persons with symptomatic MVP and the relative benefits of specific methods of nursing assistance. While these descriptive studies were rich in information, sample size limited confidence in generalizability. The next stage for this programme of studies was the development of an empirical data collection tool to gather larger quantities of specific information relevant to health deviation self-care requisite categories from the clients' perspective.

Study 4: questionnaire construction and validation

While the first three studies were conducted in north-western Ohio, the principal researcher moved to central Virginia in 1988, providing an opportunity to examine the reliability of research findings. Based on findings from previous studies, research questions were revised as the project continued in central Virginia.

The new research questions reflected the development of a data collection instrument constructed to facilitate the acquisition of data similar to that collected in studies 1 and 2. Target items on the survey instrument addressed aspects of the lived experience of MVP, specifically as based on Orem's categories of health deviation self-care requisites. Symptom experience, the relative perceived seriousness of MVP as a health problem and perceptions of treatment regimens were elicited through open- and closed-ended questions. Research questions to be addressed were:

(1) What concerns are noted by clients in the new region?
(2) Are therapeutic self-care demands similar?
(3) Do those with symptomatic MVP have similar perceptions concerning their nursing care needs?

Survey of Virginian MVP patients

Replication involves the duplication of a previous study with a new method, new sample and/or the passage of time (Burns & Grove, 1987). In this programme of studies, an earlier study was replicated in a second geographical area with a different research team. However, this replication was actually an expansion of previous studies. The method varied in that a more 'objective' instrument, derived from previous findings, was used as the data source. The testing of the new instrument involved construct validation of response items as well as checking the external validity of previous studies.

Sample

A sample of people with symptomatic MVP was obtained partially through a medical records review in a large tertiary-care centre. The study was approved by the institutional human subjects review committee and classified as 'exempt', since return of any questionnaire would be considered consent to participate. Questionnaires were mailed to those whose records included 'typical' symptoms and two-dimensional echocardiogram verification of MVP. One hundred and thirty-two surveys were sent; 38 were returned, for a rate of 29%.

To enlarge the sample and provide a community service, advertisements were placed in several university-based and local publications announcing the formation of an MVP support group. Those who responded to the advertisements were invited to attend evening information/support group meetings and also asked to complete the research instrument. Off-site completion of the questionnaire was voluntary and anonymous. Many participants in the support group expressed gratitude for the opportunity to 'tell their stories', and they were later provided with a summary of the compiled data.

The formation of the group was in an effort both to meet perceived needs for nursing service by the population of persons with MVP and to enhance the empirical knowledge of their identified needs. Thirty-eight completed and partially completed survey instruments were returned to the investigator. The sample was all female, predominantly white (92%), ranging in age from 20 to 63 ($\bar{x} = 42$).

Results

Research findings were consistent with those reported in the literature and found previously by the investigators. Responses externally validated previous studies, added evidence of construct validity for the survey instrument, and added richness to the existing data set. Once again, the overwhelming majority of respondents reported seeking health care for help with symptoms often associated with MVP, including moderate to severe chest pain, palpitations, shortness of breath, syncope and fatigue. In addition, symptoms such as tingling and numbness of extremities and sensations of circulatory changes which had been identified in study 1 and not described in the literature were again found.

The proportion of health concerns reported was much greater than the frequency of seeking care. Reported levels of attempts to follow medical regimens were high and inability to take medications was nearly always attributed to lack of effectiveness or the occurrence of troublesome side-effects. The perceived impact of symptoms on the daily life of those diagnosed with MVP was often dramatic. Results of this fourth study, therefore, validated initial findings by researchers about the specific self-care demands of persons with symptomatic MVP and their need for nursing assistance.

Summary and conclusions

Tomlinson *et al.*, (1986) have argued that programmes of research may help to maximize the benefits of research efforts and also serve to build theory. Furthermore, Fawcett & Tulman (1990) have suggested that the use of an established nursing theory framework may be helpful in selecting variables and promoting systematic examination of a clinical problem.

A series of four studies has been described in which the health and self-care needs of people with mitral valve prolapse were systematically examined by using Orem's model as a framework. This model was found to be useful used as an organizing framework, both in moving the investigators from initially vague clinical issues to clear nursing research questions, and in defining specific variables for study.

In the present series of studies, the researchers incorporated knowledge from other disciplines such as physiology and psychology: however, Orem's model aided the researchers to maintain a focus on research questions salient to nursing and to nursing practice and to build knowledge systematically in order to respond to relevant clinical issues.

Although this approach may not be applicable to all nursing research, it is one method for promoting focused building of theoretical and clinical nursing knowledge.

Acknowledgements

Funding sources for this research were as follows: studies 1 and 2 – American Nurses Foundation, for which the first author was named Burroughs Wellcome Fund Scholar; study 3 – Medical College of Ohio School of Nursing, Center for Nursing Research; study 4 – University of Virginia School of Nursing, Center for Nursing Research.

The authors wish to acknowledge the contributions of Virginia Whitmire,

PhD, RN, Susan Grass, MSN, RN, Joyce Hammer, MSN, RN, and Judy G. Ozbolt, PhD, RN.

References

Allan, J.D. & Hall, B.A. (1988) Changing the focus on technology: a critique of the medical model in a changing health care system. *ANS: Advances in Nursing Science*, **10**(3), 22–34.

Anderson, S. (1990) *Mitral Valve Prolapse: Benign Syndrome?* Videotext, Barrie, Ontario.

Burns, N. & Grove, S.K. (1987) *The Practice of Nursing Research: Conduct, Critique, and Utilization*. Saunders, Philadelphia.

Cash, J.T. & Grissett, G. (1985) Not life threatening: mitral valve prolapse syndrome. *Focus on Critical Care*, **12**(6), 54–7.

Chance, H.C. & Hinshaw, A.S. (1980) Strategies for initiating a research program. *The Journal of Nursing Administration*, **10**(3), 32–9.

Cole, F.L. & Slocumb, E.M. (1990) Collaborative nursing research between novices: productivity through partnership. *Nursing Forum*, **25**(4), 13–18.

Devereux, R.B. (1989) Diagnosis and prognosis of mitral valve prolapse. *The New England Journal of Medicine*, **320**(16), 1077–1079.

Fawcett, J. & Tulman, L. (1990) Building a programme of research from the Roy adaptation model of nursing. *Journal of Advanced Nursing*, **15**, 720–25.

Grass, S. & Utz, S.W. (1986) Mitral valve prolapse: a review of the scientific and medical literature. *Heart and Lung*, **15**(5), 507–14.

Levy, D. & Savage, D. (1987) Prevalence and clinical features of mitral valve prolapse. *American Heart Journal*, **113**(5), 1281–90.

MacMahon, S.W. Devereux, R.B. & Schron, E. (1987) Clinical and epidemiological issues in mitral valve prolapse. *American Heart Journal*, **113**(5), 1265–80.

Marks, A.R., Choong, C.Y., Sanfillipo, A.J., Ferre, M. & Weyman, A.E. (1989) Identification of high-risk and low-risk groups of patients with mitral valve prolapse. *New England Journal of Medicine*, **320**(16), 1031–6.

Orem, D.E. (1985) *Nursing: Concepts of Practice*, 3rd edn. McGraw-Hill, New York.

Orem, D. (1991) *Nursing: Concepts of Practice*, 4th edn. Mosby, St Louis.

Perloff, J.K. & Child, J.S. (1987) Clinical and epidemiological issues in mitral valve prolapse: overview and perspective. *American Heart Journal*, **113**(5), 1324–32.

Schlodtfeldt, R.M. (1986) Nursing: an academic discipline? Reflections on the past, images for the future. *Ohio Nurses' Review*, **61**(6), 6–8.

Simonetti, D. (1980) Prolapsed mitral valve: living with chest pain. *American Journal of Nursing*, **80**(8), 1430–32.

Smith, J. (1981) The idea of health: a philosophical inquiry. *Advances in Nursing Science*, **3**, 43–50.

Spradley, J.P. (1979) *The Ethnographic Interview*. Holt Rinehart & Winston, New York.

Stevenson, J.S. (1988) Nursing knowledge development: into era II. *Journal of Professional Nursing*, **4**(3), 152–62.

Tomlinson, P.S., Semradek, J.A., Duncan, M.T. & Boyd, S.T. (1986) Programmatic research: a collaborative model. *Journal of Professional Nursing*, **2**, 309–17.

Utz, S.W. & Grass, S.L. (1987) Mitral valve prolapse: self-care needs, nursing diagnoses and interventions. *Heart and Lung*, **16**(1), 77–83.

Utz, S.W., Hammer, J., Whitmire, V.M. & Grass, S.L. (1990) Perceptions of body image and health in persons with mitral valve prolapse. *Image: The Journal of Nursing Scholarship*, **22**(1), 18–22.

Williams, C.A. (1989) Establishing a research program and teaching undergraduates: are they compatible? *Journal of Professional Nursing*, **5**(2), 60.

Chapter 10
The Betty Neuman Systems Model applied to practice: a client with multiple sclerosis

JANET B. KNIGHT, *BScN, MScN, RN*
Assistant Professor, School of Nursing, University of Ottawa, Ottawa, Canada

The importance of nursing theories and models for the growth and development of the profession of nursing is widely acknowledged. The variety of nursing phenomena and situations demands some flexibility in the choice of specific conceptualizations to be used. This chapter demonstrates the goodness of fit of the Betty Neuman Systems Model to the care of clients with multiple sclerosis. An adapted assessment tool, based on Neuman's tool, but more useful in the acute care medical setting, is used to gather data related to a woman with recently diagnosed multiple sclerosis. A nursing care plan illustrating the use of Neuman's model is generated, implemented and evaluated. The Neuman model is demonstrated to be useful and effective in the implementation of the nursing process in this case.

Introduction

The 1980s have been characterized by the acceptance of the significance of theories and models for nursing (Fawcett, 1989; Meleis, 1985). Such conceptualization helps to clearly define the domain of nursing by differentiating it from the domain of medicine and other health care disciplines. They provide coherent and systematic frameworks which can guide and direct nursing assessment, planning and intervention. The language of models and theories, the definitions of terms and the descriptions of concepts, provide grounds for communication among nurses and are essential for nursing research (Fawcett, 1989; Jacox, 1974). The conceptual-theoretical system of knowledge – represented by models and theories – is a vehicle of professionalism (Gruending, 1985), especially for those professional attributes of accountability and autonomy (Fuller, 1978; McKay, 1969).

   The enormous variety of nursing phenomena and the situations in which they occur demand some flexibility in the choice of nursing theories or models as the situation dictates (McGee, 1984). This chapter describes some salient features of nursing clients with multiple sclerosis (MS), demonstrates the goodness-of-fit of the Betty Neuman Systems Model (Neuman 1989) to the care of these clients, and specifically illustrates the application of this model to a case study of a client with MS. A modified assessment tool, based on Neuman's tool, is utilized and is shown to apply to acute care medical patients.

Salient features of multiple sclerosis

Multiple sclerosis is a generally non-fatal, chronic and often progressive disease of the central nervous system which occurs primarily between the ages of 20 and 40 years. The uncertainty related to the course of the disease and the actual or potential disruption of various motor, sensory or cognitive functions, can have complex and unpredictable effects on every aspect of a person's life. The nurse caring for the client with MS must have a guide or framework for carrying out the nursing process in situations with complex and interactive variables. In MS, as in many chronic unpredictable conditions, the meanings or interpretations that the client gives to the disease and its many physical and psychosocial effects, are of critical importance in relation to the client's adjustment (Brooks & Matson, 1982; Duval, 1984). Clients with chronic disease should ideally manage their own lives and should be co-creators with nurses and others of plans to help them maintain, regain, or attain optimum functioning (McEwen *et al.*, 1983). A nursing framework that is suitable for working with clients with MS must accommodate for the importance of perception and be compatible with the collaborative approach between the client and caregiver.

MS is a disease with the possibility of remissions and exacerbations and an overall decrease in functional ability as time progresses. A useful nursing framework should accommodate for the need to prevent complications, treat acute problems and rehabilitate the client. Finally, there is so far no proven medical treatment to halt or slow the progress of this disease. This condition requires management of specific responses of the client to improve his functioning in daily life. An avoidance of the 'sick role' for these clients is essential. A nursing framework which is not dependent on the medical model or the concept of illness is essential for working with MS clients.

The fit of the Neuman Model

The Betty Neuman Systems Model is ideally suited for guiding nursing practice in relation to the client with MS. The model's open-system characteristics, its incorporation of the time variable, and its consideration of five major client variables accommodate the complexity and unpredictability of situations encountered by the MS client. The model's major focus on perception is extremely helpful for dealing with various clients' feelings, attitudes and beliefs that may affect the course of the disease and the appropriateness of management goals and modalities. The three levels of prevention in this model – primary, secondary and tertiary – certainly fit the various settings in which the client may encounter a nurse. The model's non-reliance on the medical model or the concept of illness is another reason for its adoption in the case of a client with MS.

The following section presents a brief summary of the major concepts and assumptions of the model. The model is then applied to a case study of a young woman with MS.

The Neuman Systems Model

This section describes the Neuman (1989) model in terms of the four meta-paradigms of nursing (Fawcett, 1989): person, environment, health, and nursing. For a diagrammatic conceptualization of Neuman's model see Fig. 10.1.

Person

Neuman (1989) views the client (an individual or collective entity) as an open system. The individual client is a dynamic composite of the interrelationship of five variables: physiologic, psychologic, sociocultural, spiritual and developmental. To meet personal needs, the client interacts with the envir-

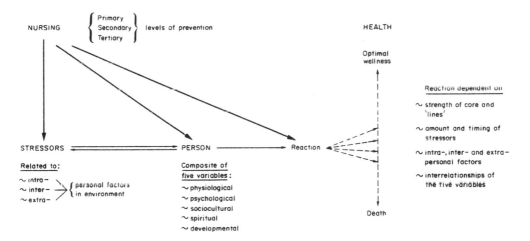

Fig. 10.1 A conceptualization of the Betty Neuman Systems Model.

onment and affects it and is affected by it. Each individual has characteristics or responses that fall within a common range and sets of strengths or specific responses that set him apart as unique.

The system of the client can be portrayed figuratively (Fig. 10.2) by a core of basic structure and energy resources surrounded by three hypothetical concentric circles representing boundaries (Neuman 1989). The closest boundary, the lines of resistance, protects the core and consists of internal defensive processes such as the immune response and physiological homeostatic mechanisms. The next boundary is the normal line of defence, or dynamic equilibrium, and represents what the person has become over time. It includes such aspects as intelligence, attitudes, and problem solving and coping abilities. The outermost boundary is the flexible line of defence, a protective buffer for the normal line of defence. It has an accordian-like action which changes in a relatively short time dependent on such factors as amount of sleep, level of nutrition, and the quality and quantity of stress.

A person is constantly subject to stressors from within his own system and from the environment which can cause disequilibrium, situational or maturational crises, disease or death (Neuman 1989). Reaction to stressors is determined in part by natural and learned resistance which is manifested by the strength of the core and the various lines. Factors which influence the reaction to stressors are intra-, inter-or extra-personal in nature. The quality and quantity of an individual's reaction to stressors is determined by the interrelationships of the five variables. Of critical importance is the person's perception of a stressor since it can affect the person's resistance and

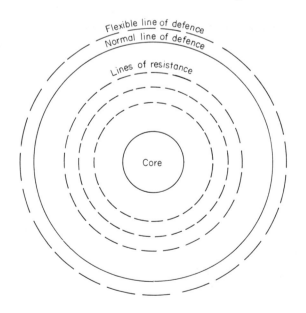

Fig. 10.2   The conception of the person in Betty Neuman's Systems Model (based on Neuman 1989).

response to the stressor. The number, timing and intensity of stressors also affect a person's resistance to a stressor.

Environment

Neuman states that the environment is 'that viable arena which has relevance to the life span of an organism' (Neuman, 1989). She also views it as all factors affecting or affected by a person. Neuman contends that there is an internal and external environment, a point which confuses many as she does not clearly delineate the boundaries between person and environment. Neuman (1989) suggests that the environment is the source of stressors and provides resources for managing these stressors. Stressors are such things as micro-organisms, a ruptured aneurysm, radiation, excessive noise, and interpersonal conflict. Resources are entities such as a functioning immunological system, good coping skills, education, strong family support, and a community health centre. Stressors can be classified as either beneficial or noxious, depending on their nature, timing, degree and potential for either ultimate positive or negative change in the person. Neuman places more emphasis on stressors than any other aspect of the environment, as is highlighted in Fig. 10.1.

Health

Neuman (1989) states that health or wellness – she uses the terms synonymously – is equated with optimal system stability. System stability is the best possible wellness state at any given time. Optimum wellness occurs when all needs are met. Conversely, illness – or variance from wellness, as she terms it – is a state of insufficiency or instability, a state in which disrupting needs are yet to be satisfied and the normal line of defence is penetrated (Neuman 1989). Confusingly, Neuman states that health is both continuous and dichotomous with wellness at one end and extreme variances from wellness (and ultimately death) at the other end. She uses the term reconstitution to describe the events which occur following the impact of a stressor. In the process of reconstruction, a person can progress beyond his normal line of defence to a higher than usual state of wellness or below his usual state of wellness.

Nursing

Nursing is defined by Neuman as a 'unique profession that is concerned with all variables affecting an individual's responses to stressors' (Neuman, 1974). The main concern of nursing is the total person and the goal of nursing is to maintain, regain or attain client system stability. Neuman suggests that this stability or maximum level of wellness can be attained 'by purposeful interventions ... aimed at reduction of stress factors and adverse conditions which either affect or could affect optimal functioning in a given client situation' (Neuman, 1982).

Nursing process

Neuman's (1989) process contains three basic parts: nursing diagnosis, nursing goals, and nursing outcomes. Neuman stresses the importance of identifying client and caregiver perceptions and collaborating between client and caregiver at all stages of the process. Table 10.1 summarizes Neuman's nursing process steps.

Levels of prevention

Neuman (1989) states that intervention can begin at any point at which the stressor is suspected or detected and identified. Based on the time frame associated with the stressor impact on the person, Neuman has developed three levels of prevention. Primary prevention is selected when a stressor is suspected but no reaction has taken place. Intervention strategies include education, desensitization against risks, avoidance of hazards, and strengthening resistance to risks. Secondary prevention is appropriate when a reaction to a stressor has already occurred. At this level the caregiver

Table 10.1   Summary of Betty Neuman's nursing process steps.

A. Nursing diagnosis
1. *Data base and assessment*
   - identification, classification, and evaluation of interactions among five client variables.
   - identification of stressors and resources in the intra-, inter- and extra-personal areas.
   - identification and differentiation of client and caregiver perceptions.
   - attempt to resolve perceptual differences.
2. *Actual or potential variances from wellness*
   (These are what most other theorists call 'nursing diagnoses'.)

B. Nursing goals
1. *Expected outcomes*, i.e. specific desirable behavioural responses to deal with the actual or potential variances from wellness (decided by client and caregiver in collaboration).
2. *Planned interventions*, i.e. specific actions of client, caregiver or others to affect outcomes.

C. Nursing outcomes
1. *Actual interventions*, i.e. interventions actually carried out.
2. *Evaluation and goal reformulation*
   - analysis of specific client responses.
   - determination of attainment of expected outcomes.
   - if incomplete attainment, determination of cause of non-attainment.
   - goal reformulation as needed.

---

prioritizes the client's needs and carries out actions aimed at stabilizing the system by conserving client energy or purposefully manipulating stressors or reaction to stressors. Tertiary prevention is used after some interventions at the secondary level prevention have been instituted and some degree of reconstitution has occurred. Tertiary level interventions include increasing motivation, modifying maladaptive behaviour, orienting to reality, or re-education.

Application of the Neuman Model

Client profile

Miss T. is a 22-year-old third-year university student who is engaged to be married but plans to finish her degree in physical education first. She has been in excellent health until recently. She was hospitalized for investigation of the third episode in a period of five months of weakness and numbness in her legs. During her admission neurological assessment, it was noted that she had decreased motor coordination on her right side, slight lack of equilibrium, some mild weakness in both legs, and nystagmus. She reported 'seeing double', some numbness in her right leg, and some urinary urgency and frequency. She displayed signs of mild anxiety. She reported that she had been to the doctor several times in the past two years because of dizziness, excessive fatigue and several minor musculoskeletal complaints. About six months ago her physician suggested that there was nothing organically wrong and that she was experiencing a stress reaction. Counselling was advised but she did not follow through with the doctor's suggestion.

At the start of this case study, Miss T. has been in the hospital for eight days and had had blood, urine and cerebrospinal fluid tests, skull and spinal X-rays, computerized axial tomography and magnetic resonance imaging scans, an electroencephalogram, and visual and auditory evoked potentials. All of the investigations were normal except for her cerebrospinal fluid tests which revealed elevated total protein, elevated gamma globulin and oligoclonal bands. The neurologist informed her that these results were highly suggestive of MS.

Assessment tool

The following tool was used to gather data about Miss T. by the nurse. Based on Neuman's (1989) tool, it has been adapted by the author and her colleagues to more readily fit an acute care medical setting. There are two areas of change. Section A, the intake summary, has been expanded to include data about diagnosis, admission and discharge, medication and other pertinent facts. Section D1a, the physiological section of intra-personal factors, has been expanded to include a system review and a two item functional review. These additions constitute a minor adaptation of Neuman's instrument and in no way affect the application of the model itself.

A. Intake summary

(1) Name
(2) Age
(3) Marital status
(4) Medical diagnosis
(5) Date of admission to hospital
(6) Date of discharge from hospital
(7) Date of assessment
(8) Other pertinent facts
(9) Medications

B. Stressors (as perceived by client)

(1) What do you consider your major problem, stress area or areas of concern?
(2) How do present circumstances differ from your usual pattern of living?
(3) Have you ever experienced a similar problem? If so, what was the problem and how did you handle it? Were you successful?
(4) What do you anticipate for yourself in the future as a consequence of your present situation?
(5) What are you doing and what can you do to help yourself?
(6) What do you expect caregivers, family, friends or others to do for you?

C. Stressors (as perceived by the nurse)

The same six questions, as above, should be answered, but from the standpoint of how the *nurse* evaluates the client, the client's major problem, pattern of living, present and past coping strategies, and expectations for the future and of others.

D. Summary of impressions

(1) Intrapersonal factors
(a) Physiological
System review:
Neurological
Gastrointestinal

Respiratory
Genito-urinary
Musculoskeletal
Cardiovascular
Dermatological
Endocrine-reproductive
Functional status:
Activities of daily living
Rest and sleep
  (b) Psychological
  (c) Sociocultural
  (d) Developmental
  (e) Spiritual
(2) *Interpersonal factors*
Resources, relationships of family, friends, caregivers
(3) *Extrapersonal factors*
Resources, relationships with other groups, institutions, financial, employment

E. Formulation of actual or potential variances from wellness (nursing diagnoses)

Assessment findings

A. Intake summary

  (1) Name: Miss T.
  (2) Age: Female
  (3) Marital status: Single
  (4) Medical diagnosis: Probable MS
  (5) Date of admission to hospital: 15 February
  (6) Date of discharge: (still hospitalized)
  (7) Date of assessment(s): 15–23 February
  (8) Other pertinent facts
  (9) Medications: Multivitamins and birth control pills

B. Client's perception of stressors

Miss T.'s major concern was the meaning that the diagnosis of MS has in relation to her plans for finishing her degree, a career in physical education, marriage, and a family. Her immediate area of stress was how she was going to make up classes and assignments. She had always been very physically active and was proud that she was strong, physically fit and as 'healthy as a horse'. She had a recurrent mental image of the only person she knows with

MS, an incontinent, partially blind wheelchair-bound man. She declared 'I'm not going to give in to this! I will be better if I just get back to my usual regime of physical activity and my well balanced diet.' She expected the neurologist to discuss aspects of neuropathology and possible treatment with her. She thought the nurses could help her by answering some questions about MS, 'but the nurses seem so busy; I have to bother them'. She said 'My parents are really upset by this. I've got to put on a brave face' and 'My fiancé is such a support for me, I don't know what I would do without him'.

C. Nurse's perceptions of stressors

Miss T.'s major stressor was the profound threat that this recent altered functioning and diagnosis of probable MS has had to her image of herself as physically fit, strong and possessing mastery over the functioning of her body. A secondary, but important stressor was the threat to present and future roles as student, career woman, wife and mother. The stressor of the inflammatory process in her nervous system was important but, beyond the use of corticosteroids, there is no known direct way to influence this process, more than temporarily.

She had never had a similar crisis before and her coping style at the time of the case study was a combination of information seeking, intellectualizing, and some denial of the seriousness of the diagnosis and her need for emotional support. She constantly asked several different nurses the same questions. Her affect varied between cheerfulness and seeming unconcern and some withdrawal and agitation. She was sleeping poorly, but resisted attempts by the nurses to discuss her concerns. She was very anxious to get back to her apartment so she would have more control over her life. She relied almost exclusively on her fiancé for emotional support and seemed to expect very little of any of the health professionals, friends or her parents. Although Miss T.'s strengths of intelligence, knowledge (related to diet, exercise and fitness), and self-reliance would certainly be assets in dealing with the stressors, it appeared that if she did not acknowledge her need for emotional support and exploration of her feelings with appropriate resource people, she might not be able to handle the crisis.

D. Summary of impressions (only significant findings are noted here)

    (1) Intrapersonal factors
        (a) Physiological
            System review
            Neurological – left eye lagging on abduction, reports intermittent diplopia; horizontal nystagmus with slight right and left lateral gaze;

inability to tandem walk; falls to right during Rhomberg test; slight slowness and clumsiness of right arm during rapidly alternating movements; difficulty with moving right heel down left shin; slight weakness in hip flexors.

Gastrointestinal – none.

Respiratory – respiratory rate 28, frequent sighing; non-smoker.

Genito-urinary – reports urinary frequency intermittently over past year.

Musculoskeletal – well-developed muscles and except for above noted abnormalities, exhibits above average strength in most muscle groups of arms and legs.

Cardiovascular – apical rate 92.

Dermatological – none.

Endocrine-reproductive – on birth control pills for three years; yearly normal pap smears.

Functional status

Activities of daily living – reports intermittent mild to severe fatigue over three years, worse in past year; has had to cut out extra-curricular sports (volleyball and tennis) this term. Managing with effort to meet her academic requirements. Difficulty in doing her share of household chores.

Rest and sleep – unable to rest and sleep adequately in hospital environment; walks around ward and hospital during day; has difficulty sitting still or resting; sleeps six to seven hours at night with frequent waking; refuses oxazepam ordered as sedative.

b. Psychological

Mood labile (see stressors as perceived by nurse); would not talk in any depth about her feelings about the diagnosis; was unhappy that she could not maintain her usual diet (high fibre, low animal fat, avoidance of refined carbohydrates) in the hospital; spent a lot of time with her fiancé and was frequently seen quietly crying while in discussion with him.

c. Sociocultural

Is a member of mainstream white Anglo-Saxon cultural group; strong belief system which values education, self-reliance, working hard, and physical strength and fitness; values women having equal status with men in all areas.

d. Developmental

Has been successfully engaged in meeting developmental needs appropriate to a young adult, i.e. preparing for a career and marriage.

e. Spiritual

Considers herself a Christian, but has not regularly attended church since she left home for university; stated she talks to her fiancé and others about religious and ethical beliefs but does not feel comfortable with organized religion.

(2) Interpersonal factors

Miss T. is an only child. Her parents are healthy and live 50 miles away. She feels respect and affection for her parents, but considers herself to be largely independent of them. She and her fiancé are close and mutually supportive. They have lived together for a year and have several friends in common, mostly other couples. She has two close women friends, but her contact with them has decreased since her engagement a year ago. Her fiancé has stated to several nurses that since Miss T.'s hospitalization he has felt a lot of stress, has had headaches and abdominal pain, and has had difficulty in keeping up with his graduate school work in biomedical engineering. Miss T. has not relied on nursing or medical staff for more than straightforward discussions of 'facts' related to diagnostic tests and to MS.

(3) Extrapersonal factors

Miss T. is on a scholarship which provides for tuition, books, supplies and partial housing allowance. She uses student loans and summer employment to provide money for housing, clothes, food and other expenses. Medical insurance is covered by student fees at her university so hospitalization and doctors' visits are covered. The university has an excellent student health service which includes provision for counselling. There is a large and active MS Society in Miss T.'s community which holds nurse-led self-help groups for the newly diagnosed.

E. Actual or potential variances from wellness (nursing diagnoses)

(1) Disturbance in self-concept due to mild decrease in muscle strength, co-ordination and overall stamina, and to recent medical diagnosis of MS.

(2) Potential for ineffective coping with and adjustment to diagnosis of MS and altered physical functioning due to (i) fear of dependence, loss of autonomy, lack of fulfilment of academic occupational and personal/social goals, and (ii) her exhausting the emotional resources of her fiancé.

(3) Knowledge deficit related to lack of experience and facts related to MS, including its signs and symptoms, prognosis, course, role of attitudes and emotions, management and resources.

(4) Mild alteration in mobility, coordination and stamina due to MS.

Short-term nursing goals

The nurse shared her diagnoses with Miss T. and in general Miss T. accepted them, although she did not feel comfortable with 'the potential for ineffective coping' despite being willing to explore the possibility. Miss T. and the nurse negotiated some short-term goals. The following section outlines the expected outcomes and planned interventions that comprised nursing goals to address each of the four nursing diagnoses.

1. Related to diagnosis 1

A. Expected outcomes

(1) Miss T. will verbalize an acceptance of the idea that she may have to redefine the parameters of her highly valued self-concepts of strength, fitness, autonomy (within four days).

(2) Miss T. will verbalize a continued motivation, within the limitations of her strength and energy, to maintain activities which will maintain her present high level of fitness and general strength (ongoing).

B. Planned interventions (combined primary and secondary level prevention)

(1) Daily sessions (of at least 30 minutes) with the nurse in a quiet private room to explore: Miss T.'s feelings about the diagnosis, her symptoms, the meanings the disease has for her and possible modifications of her expectations and activities.

(2) Reinforcement by the nurse of Miss T.'s appropriate use of the nursing staff for emotional support and explorations of feelings and attitudes.

(3) Exploration of acceptability to Miss T. of a referral to the MS Society – to talk to another person with MS on the telephone, in person, or as a member of a group for the newly diagnosed.

2. Related to diagnosis 2

A. Expected outcomes

(1) Miss T. will continue to discuss openly that there is a good possibility of ineffective coping with the diagnosis and altered functioning if she does not deal with her fear of loss of her autonomy and lack of fulfilment of academic, occupational and personal goals (ongoing).

(2) Miss T. will list other potential resources to supply emotional support and temporary assistance with domestic chores (shopping, cooking, cleaning) and academic requirements upon her discharge from the hospital (three days).

(3) Miss T. will identify alternate short-term adjustments to her course load and extra-curricular activities (three days).

B. Planned interventions (primary level prevention)

(1) Daily sessions (concurrent with 1.B.1 above) to discuss fears, alternative resources and short-term coping strategies.

(2) Referral to community health nurse upon discharge to follow up on discussion of fears, resources and coping strategies.

(3) If required, liaison by nurse or Miss T. with academic counsellor to explore feasibility of adjustment of academic requirements.

3. Related to diagnosis 3

A.

(1) Miss T. can explain the very basic facts about the pathology of MS, the basis of her own symptoms, the highly variable course of the disease, the importance of attention to emotional health, and any other areas about which she expresses curiosity (by discharge).

(2) Miss T. verbalizes and demonstrates coping strategies for management of her present problems with fatigue, decreased muscle strength, slight incoordination and intermittent diplopia (four days or by discharge).

(3) Miss T. can list reliable and questionable resources for more information about MS and its management.

B. Planned interventions (combined primary and secondary level prevention)

(1) Ongoing informal instruction and answering Miss T.'s questions on MS and its management.

(2) Considering Miss T.'s readiness and appropriateness of specific material, provision of information booklets about MS.

(3) If acceptable referral to the MS Society as a source of reliable information.

4. Related to diagnosis 4

A. Expected outcomes

(1) Miss T. will demonstrate and explain methods to manage her:
   (a) decreased muscle strength (mostly right leg);
   (b) slight incoordination/lack of balance;
   (c) fatigue; and
   (d) intermittent diplopia. (By three days.)

B. Planned interventions (examples of primary and secondary level preventions)

(1) The nurse will discuss and/or demonstrate management strategies for:
   (a) decreased muscle strength, e.g. (1) active exercise within limits of fatigue, with periodic rest periods; (2) avoidance of very long and heavy periods of exercise.
   (b) slight incoordination/lack of balance, e.g. (1) avoidance of hazardous activities requiring good coordination; (2) tub baths instead of showers; (3) avoidance of quick turning; (4) low heeled shoes.

(c) fatigue, e.g. (1) pacing and timing of activities to avoid overexertion; (2) daily rest periods; (3) sitting instead of standing when possible.

(d) diplopia, e.g. (1) patching of one eye; (2) avoidance of eye muscle strain.

Nursing outcomes

The following is a summary of actual interventions, evaluation and goal reformulation after one week.

1. *Related to diagnosis 1*

Two nurses, Mrs B. and Miss A., developed a close therapeutic relationship with Miss T. She became much more honest about her feelings, crying openly at times and expressing some anger that such a thing should happen to her. She expressed some grief that she may have to adjust her self-concept to incorporate the new fact of 'probably MS'. She verbalized that perhaps she will have to focus now on 'other ways of being strong'. She is cautiously optimistic that she can manage not to push herself too much when she is discharged. She met a 30-year-old woman, Mrs Z. (another patient), who has had MS for five years and functions very well. They have had many long discussions and Miss T. appears to have been very encouraged by this woman's example. (Expected outcomes met.)

2. *Related to diagnosis 2*

Miss T. stated she realizes how difficult her illness has been for her fiancé. She is worried that he may not be able to cope with all of the present and future problems. Seeing his distress has made her feel more frightened and upset. She realizes her difficulty in sharing her feelings with people other than her fiancé. She fears her overdependence on him may backfire onto her if she does not seek other sources of help. Mrs Z. has reinforced to Miss T. how important it was to her to talk about her anger, fear and sadness with people outside her family and especially with other people with MS. Mrs Z. was discharged and she and Miss T. have talked on the phone and plan to see each other when Miss T. is discharged.

Miss T. and her fiancé have decided that when she is discharged he will do major shopping and some cleaning and that they will share cooking responsibilities. It may be necessary to have a cleaning agency in once every two weeks. She wants to have some extended discussions with a professional after discharge to discuss important concerns related to her career, marriage and family plans, and will call the student counselling service at the university. She is still quite worried about catching up with her academic work, but cannot at this time envision what adjustments could be made. The referral to the community health nurse has been made and Miss T. is happy to have this follow through.

(Comment: expected outcomes 1 and 2 met. The third, related to identifying adjustments to her academic and extracurricular activities, cannot be dealt with now.)

3. Related to diagnosis 3 and diagnosis 4

Miss T. seems to have a good basic understanding of MS and her knowledge of anatomy and physiology have helped her grasp the pathological basis for her own signs and symptoms. She has read some very basic pamphlets on MS but states she just cannot read too much more now. 'Some of it is too depressing'. She understands that MS is highly variable in its course and that it is impossible to make any predictions about an individual's prognosis. She wanted to discuss more about how she felt about the disease and what she could do to manage the specific difficulties she was experiencing. She readily accepted the proposed strategies for dealing with her specific problems. Her diplopia and fatigue appeared improved; her other problems persisted but were adequately managed by the proposed interventions. Miss T. knows about the MS Society and would like to receive some literature from them. She is not sure she wants any direct contact with the people in the Society at this time. (Expected outcomes met.)

Miss T.'s nurses and the discharge planning nurse are working on longer term goals that relate to Miss T.'s adjustment to having a serious illness with an uncertain future.

Conclusion

The Betty Neuman Systems Model (Neuman 1989) has been applied to the case of a young woman recently diagnosed as having MS. Miss T. has experienced several stressors: the process which initiates inflammation in the white matter of the central nervous system; the resulting host of minor but disturbing dysfunctions which interfere with her daily life; a diagnosis of serious disease; and a threat to her self-concept, her body image and to her present and future roles. Miss T.'s flexible line of defence has not been able to prevent the penetration of her normal line of defence.

An adapted tool suitable for use in acute care medical settings was applied. Through its use, careful assessment and evaluation of Miss T.'s and the caregiver's perceptions of the various stressors and resources for coping were made and diagnoses and goals were formulated. Interventions at the primary and secondary levels of prevention were planned and implemented. In general these interventions aimed: to prevent further stressor invasions; to maintain or strengthen Miss T.'s resources; to educate her about new coping strategies, resources and information about her disease; and to conserve her energy. Finally, the outcomes of the plan were evaluated and found to be largely congruent with the expected outcomes.

References

Brooks, N. & Matson, R. (1982) Social-psychological adjustment to multiple sclerosis. *Social Science and Medicine*, **16**, 2129–35.

Duval, M. (1984) Psychosocial metaphors of physical distress among MS patients. *Social Science and Medicine*, **19**, 635–8.

Fawcett, J. (1989) *Analysis and Evaluation of Conceptual Models of Nursing*, 2nd edn. F.A. Davis, Philadelphia.

Fuller, S. (1978) Holistic man and the science and practice of nursing. *Nursing Outlook*, **26**, 700–704.

Gruending, D. (1985) Nursing theory: a vehicle of professionalization? *Journal of Advanced Nursing*, **10**, 553–8.

Jacox, A. (1974) Theory construction in nursing: an overview. *Nursing Research*, **23**, 4–13.

McEwen, J., Martini, C. & Wilkins, N. (1983) *Participation in Health*. Croom Helm, London.

McGee, M. (ed.) (1984) *Theoretical Pluralism in Nursing Science*. University of Ottawa Press, Ottawa.

McKay, R. (1969) Theories, models and systems for nursing, *Nursing Research*, **18**, 393–9.

Meleis, A. (1985) *Theoretical Nursing*. J.B. Lippincott, London.

Neuman, B. (1974) The Betty Neuman health-care systems model: a total person approach to patient problems. In *Conceptual Models for Nursing Practice* (eds. J. Riehl & C. Roy), pp. 119–31. Appleton–Century–Crofts, New York.

Neuman, B. (1982) *The Neuman Systems Model: Application to Nursing Education and Practice*. Appleton–Century–Crofts, Norwalk, Connecticut.

Neuman, B. (1989) *The Neuman Systems Model*. Appleton and Lange, Norwalk, Connecticut.

Chapter 11
The ageing family in crisis: assessment and decision-making models

ANN C. BECKINGHAM, *RN, PhD*

Professor, School of Nursing, Educational Centre for Ageing and Health

and ANDREA BAUMANN, *RN, PhD*

Professor, School of Nursing, Faculty of Health Sciences, McMaster University, Hamilton, Ontario, Canada

This chapter presents a multidisciplinary model for use with elderly families in crisis and decision making. The application of systems in family assessment theory is outlined in order to understand the complexities of family assessment and decision making. A schematic family assessment and decision-making model is discussed. These models identify what the problem is, the family structure and supports, and possible interventions and evaluation. Ineffective processing strategies such as regression and premature closure are reviewed, and strategies for effective decision making are outlined.

Introduction

The purpose of this chapter is to present an assessment and decision-making model for use with elderly families in crisis situations. The models described provide a framework for the assessment and decision making of families in a systematic fashion when such crises do occur. Each person regardless of age, is affected by decisions, whether these are decisions he or she makes or whether they are decisions including other persons or family members. Health professionals can then assist the families in making a decision which they may be ill prepared for.

Making a decision can be a relatively simple process involving a straightforward issue, or it can be a very complex process. There may be many persons involved and the factors taken into account are numerous, complex, interacting, and the issue being addressed is far-reaching in scope. In this context, it is important to understand what a family is, to identify the crisis they face, and the system where interactions and decision making take place.

As people age there are many challenges as well as enriching experiences. 'As a person gets older' crises such as the need to change living arrangements, financial problems, and the inability to perform self-care activities are ubiquitous events among the very old (Kulys, 1983). Thus, the ageing family demonstrates some unique crisis situations.

A crisis may be defined as a sudden unanticipated or unplanned for event which necessitates immediate action to resolve the problem. The following crisis scenarios act as examples:

(1) A widowed woman aged 85, living alone, has to decide whether to move to Vancouver to live with her son or be institutionalized. The long-term care facility has phoned to say there is a placement for her.
(2) Evelyn has two children and a full-time position working shifts in the local store. For the past two years she has tried to visit her 76 year old uncle who lives alone, two to three times per week. On her last visit two days ago, a visiting nurse tells her that her uncle is malnourished and is spending too much time in bed.
(3) Jane has just had a telephone call at work from the head nurse on B-4 saying that she must make arrangements to taker her 90-year-old mother home tomorrow. Jane's mother has been a patient in the medical centre for three months.

It is important for nurses to identify crisis scenarios in their own clinical practice. This identification is followed by an examination of the family constellation, a family assessment, as well as a decision-making process to select and prioritize problems and carry out possible interventions.

Families in crises

A large area of debate as families and their functions change, is around the definition of family. A family has been defined by many authors, each with various interpretations. The working definition of a family can be broad, encompassing both the traditional nuclear and expanded family, the single parent and his/her social network, and the group of non-related persons living together carrying out family duties and responsibilities.

For the purpose of this chapter, family is defined as 'a group of people – often but not necessarily related by blood or marriage with a commitment to live with and care for one another over time' (Christie-Seely, 1984). This definition is congruent with that of the World Health Organization (WHO) which states: 'One person or a group of people living together and related to one another by blood, marriage or adoption' (Hogarth, 1978). In summary, one can say a family is a system composed of parts that interact in a given environment. Understanding systems theory is basic to both the family-oriented approach and the approach using the family as a decision-making unit (Egan & Cowan, 1979; Gillis *et al.*, 1989; Phillips, 1976).

Some families may manage well on their own with the above crises. Other families may experience a great sense of need, but hesitate to ask for help for fear of losing their independence or self-esteem. There are few studies that document how the very old anticipate crisis (Kulys, 1983). Families meeting the impact of illness, changing relationships or other crises can profit from external professional help especially during the acute phase of crises when the situation encountered is new and stressful. The family may need knowledge and preparation to interact successfully with the specialized, fragmented and complex health care system.

The use of a model for family assessment and decision making by nurses assists families to recognize their decision-making style when making decisions under less than ideal circumstances. Effective decision making examines as many factors as possible and results in less trial and error. Health care workers, by understanding the process of decision making, can strengthen interim coping mechanisms and assist families to review as many potential alternatives and outcomes as possible. If the focus is on the family as a system, this will assist in a more holistic recognition of a family's problems and coping mechanisms.

Families experience crises in much the same way as individuals. The nurse's role is one which helps families recognize both their independence and interdependencies in a crisis situation. Initially, it may not be the problem alone that creates the crisis, but the state of helplessness or inability to move productively toward resolution with the resultant dysphoria that accompanies the distress. A family resolves a crisis by changing itself, its situation, or both.

Crisis theorists have indicated that there is a critical time frame for intervention in crisis. It should be during the period of acute disequilibrium or after impact when the situation is most acute, and before inadequate coping patterns are established. A family assessment is the first step in the decision-making process in order to provide a compensatory evaluation of the dynamics that may exist in individual situations.

A family assessment model

Many different models or a combination of models are available for family assessment which incorporate systems and decision-making theory. The Neuman Systems Model (Neuman, 1974, 1989) as well as the Calgary Family Assessment Model (CFAM) (Wright & Leahey, 1984) provide systematic methods of assessing families (Fig. 11.1). Reed, in her chapter on the 'Neuman Systems Model: a basis for family psychosocial assessment and intervention', applies the model as a systems approach to family problems (Reed, 1989).

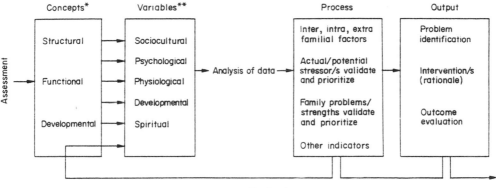

Fig. 11.1   Systems model of family assessment. *Wright & Leahey (1984); **Neuman (1982).

According to Reed, the flexible line of defence in a family can be thought of as containing variables which are found in the functional concepts of family theory. Functional concepts can be defined as variables which are used to maintain the family as an operational unit. These variables represent the dynamic state of the family as it manages the ongoing encounter with stressors. Inside the flexible line of defence is the normal line of defence. In a family, the model's normal line of defence contains the variables which are found within the structural concepts of family theory. Structural concepts are defined as variables used to provide a framework for the family system. In a family assessment, the concept of nonsummativity, or 'the whole being greater than the sum of its parts' is very important. The energy of individual members combined is greater than the energy of each individual separately. Once combined, the energy cannot be separated into parts without a change in the structure as a whole. Structural concepts may be concerned with the broad categories of communication patterns, decision-making mechanisms, mechanisms for meeting family members' needs for intimacy and affection, and ways for dealing with loss and change.

The next section of Neuman's structure is the flexible lines of resistance. In a family, the lines of resistance are comprised of concepts which protect both the family as a system, and the individuals who make up the family. The lines of resistance protect against stressors which break through the normal coping mechanisms employed by a family. They are internal factors which are used to stabilize a family and return that family to a normal coping status.

The CFAM is based on system, cybernetic and communication concepts. It consists of three major categories: family structural, developmental and functional assessment, each containing several subcategories which may be explored as appropriate to each individual family. The integration of these two complementary models, the CFAM and the Neuman Systems Model, provides one method of family assessment.

It is possible for more than one stressor to occur at a given time causing a reaction in the family system. These factors or responses may be intrafamilial (forces occurring within the family), interfamilial (forces occurring between one or more families) or extrafamilial (forces occurring outside the family). The appropriate interrelationship of these factors will determine the amount of resistance the family has to any stressor.

When analysing the family data, the assessor should identify family strengths and problems in the structural, developmental and functional categories, along with the appropriate variables. A problem/strengths list is a useful working tool. Family strengths are very important to note; some can be used effectively as interventions. Strengths such as the ability to communicate thoughts and feelings effectively, the ability to perform family roles flexibly and the ability to use a crisis experience as a means of growth, will enhance family life. Family strengths are found in the capacity to care, to share, to sacrifice, to love, to trust and to be intimate. The family is an emotional buffer between the individual and the impersonal stressful society we live in. Leavitt (1982) refers to family strengths (binding characteristics) such as stability, familiarity, love, pride and a shared identity as qualities that make a family system work for the continued health and strength of the system.

Following a family assessment the interviewer will integrate and record the assessment data in an organized format. Analysis of the data will indicate if there are problems or a crisis situation that require intervention and use of the decision-making model.

The decision-making model

Along with the family assessment model, a comprehensive decision-making model has been developed in order to provide a structure to guide health professionals in identifying factors that may impede optimum decision making.

As outlined in the following systems decision-making model (Fig. 11.2), some of the steps include:

(1) Assess and collect base-line data using the systems model of family assessment (Fig. 11.1).
(2) Examine the processing strategies.
(3) Analyse assessment data.
(4) Review the alternatives.

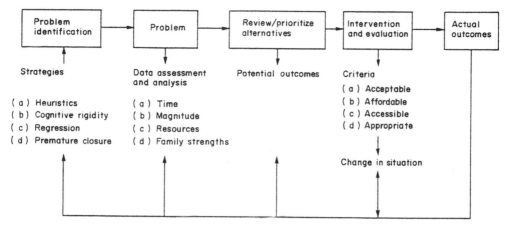

Fig. 11.2   Decision-making model in family crisis.

(5) List and prioritize all possible decisions that could be undertaken using criteria (acceptable, affordable, accessible).

(6) Implement the priority decision to reach a resolution.

(7) Evaluate.

The systems model that is presented in Fig. 11.2 indicates a series of steps where one examines and identifies a problem, reviews alternatives, carries out interventions and evaluates outcomes. Much has been written about long-term decision making assumed to be optimal because of the time allowed and people available to make the decision. In a very short period of time when a crisis is imminent, a family as a unit can be called upon to make many important decisions. There is a paucity of research about how the very old and their families anticipate and deal with the crises of ageing.

Decision-making behaviour in crisis

There is documentation on the decision-making process in clinical situations where health care providers work with older patients (Kulys, 1983; Levkoff & Wetle, 1989). The ideal decision-making process is one where people correctly identify the problem, examine and weigh alternatives and freely make a choice (Coulton *et al.*, 1988). However, in crisis, habitual patterns of decision making may not be appropriate. Crisis decision making is characterized by high risk, short decision-making time and increased stress (Holsti, 1978). The condensed time frame of a crisis situation further complicates this decision-making process. This may result in sub-optimal decision making because there is not enough time to carry out all the necessary decision-making steps. Simon (1957) has introduced the notion of 'bounded rationality', suggesting that to compensate for information over-load, the decision maker reduces a problem to a simplified representation of the problem. Rather than seeking an optimal solution, the decision maker 'satisfies' by choosing the first solution which meets the desired objectives (March & Simon, 1958). As a result, in crisis situations, individuals may rush into alternatives that would not have been their choice under better circumstances (Coulton *et al.*, 1988).

Families in crisis may have neither the time nor the experience to approach a situation using a step-by-step rational decision-making approach. In a study completed by Baumann & Bourbonnais (1984), the factors that nurses identified as important in decision making were knowledge and experiences with the problem. In many health care situations, families are exposed to unfamiliar situations where there are, in many cases, no prescribed solutions, and they are pressured to make important decisions. They need to effectively condense and utilize a great deal of information in a short period of time. In order to try and understand a problem (the first step in the decision-making process), and propose solutions, it has been documented that people use simple but misleading processing strategies (heuristics) to reduce the complexity of decision making.

Case-related information is crucial; attempts to create generic solutions without careful attention to context are likely to flounder (Deber & Baumann, 1992). This is why a systematic approach is very important in assisting families at a time when they will have a reduced ability to examine the situation and all the parameters. A clinician may assist in providing information of a very concrete nature in order to alleviate initial anxiety. The family requires assistance in not only identifying problems but anticipating what to expect and what decision strategies may be effective (Baumann, 1991). In decision-making, accurate problem identification is the most important step. If the problem is not correctly identified all subsequent steps may be invalid. Decision-making under crisis is never optimal; however, the understanding of the factors that play a role in impacting the decision is essential.

Coping with crisis

Kahneman *et al.* (1982) demonstrated that people consistently violated principles of rational decision making when they were asked to make pre-dictions or cope with probabilistic tasks. Heuristics such as 'availability' (ease of recall of past data) lead people to apply past information to present situations that may not be applicable. Although the use of heuristics in crisis situations has not been experimentally demonstrated, it can be observed in families as they try to relate this situation to a neighbour's experience or one that happened in the past to their own family. Once recognized by the nurse, families can be assisted to see what it is about this situation that is unique and what may have possible parallels with the past. Erroneous information can be excluded and only the most relevant information should be retained for the purpose of making a decision.

To further complicate matters, Holsti (1978) hypothesizes that in crisis there is not only increased reliance on past experience, but a cognitive rigidity that results in decreased span of attention and intolerance for ambiguity. The decreased attention span can be observed by families requiring information to be repeated over a period of time in the same format. The intolerance for ambiguity and a decreased sensitivity to others' perspectives is demonstrated often by the family's desire for the one right answer and wish for an immediate solution. Regressive behaviour is evident by people demonstrating confusion or anger with the health care system, verbalizing that 'they don't tell me anything'. This syndrome can be a result of the system or it can also be demonstrative of people under stress and having difficulty attending to information that is given to them.

Dubeau *et al.*, (1986) also documented premature closure which can lead to errors in problem formulation. Premature closure is when 'unjustified inferences or conclusions are drawn' before data collection is complete (Dubeau *et al.*, 1986). In a crisis, people do not take the time to examine the data which are available; they come to a conclusion before weighing all of the necessary factors.

These misleading processing strategies may inhibit accurate examination of what exactly are the actual problems. For example, in scenario 3, it would initially appear that Jane's problem is that she has to take her 90-year-old mother home tomorrow. However, using the family assessment tool one might identify related or underlying problems in the long-term relationship between Jane and her mother. This unresolved tension may impede communication and decision making about possible future alternatives. Jane has several difficult decisions to make in a short period of time. Decision making can be enhanced by assisting Jane and her mother to become focused on the most salient problem and to review the various alternatives in a systematic way.

What the nurse brings to the situation is past experience with similar situations and a knowledge base about potential problems, possible interventions and knowledge of community resources. There are strategies such as outlining, clarifying or focusing the client on the issues, which reduce the uncertainty and allow for close examination of the complexity of the problems (Baumann, 1991).

Problem identification is enhanced by analysing the assessment data, taking into consideration factors such as time, resources, magnitude of the problem, and family strengths as well as decision-making behaviour under crisis. The framework for this analysis is contained in the systems model and includes criteria for intervention, such as acceptable, affordable, accessible and appropriate, concepts of primary health care we believe are important. These indicate that the family may require information about the normal ageing process and types and range of community services that are available in order to make alternative choices (Beckingham & Du Gas, 1993).

Concepts of ageing and the family

The family system is the primary articulator of health needs across the life span of individual family members, and should participate more actively in the decision-making process (Halm, 1992). In the decision-making process, families must guard against paternalism, usurping the aged individual's ability to participate in the problem formulation and resolution. Wiley (1983) refers to 'disability within the family context' and goes on to state that disability is an unscheduled crisis which can be considered as an event related to the structure or form of a system, and an opportunity for change. He suggests that support and education as interventions may be sufficient for some families, but may not address the difficulties of many others. Clark, (1987, 1988) discusses a structure providing the base for designing interventions to enhance the quality of life, promote autonomy and personal empowerment of the elderly. Proactive strategies to plan for potential health crises and clarify personal and familial values should focus on the interdependence of generations.

In the elderly, the psychological processes required for decision making and remembering are intertwined with those for learning. Reaching a decision requires the utilization of information stored in memory as well as information currently being received from the environment. If there is noticeable loss of abilities to make rapid decisions, to learn and to retrieve information from memory, these can have deleterious effects on an individual's self-esteem, confidence and sense of well-being regardless of the cause (Fozard & Costa, 1983). The older person and their caregivers (Thompson *et al.*, 1993) should participate to the maximum extent in every decision that involves his or her physical and socio-emotional well-being. Otherwise, the very process of family decision making becomes another arena of loss for the older person.

Clients and families who are well informed and assisted to be active participants in the decision-making process may decide to do something the health professional does not like or approve of. In the long run, patients and families will do what they decide, not what we decide; better that their decisions be informed and a participatory activity, rather than destructive and painful reactivity.

References

Baumann, A.O. (1991) ALS – Decision making under uncertainty: a positive approach. *AXONE*, 40–42.

Baumann, A.S. & Bourbonnais, F.F. (1984) *Rapid Decision Making in Crisis Situations. A Case Study Approach for Nurses*. McGraw-Hill Ryerson, Toronto.

Beckingham, A.C. & Du Gas, B. (1993) *Promoting healthy aging: a musing and commentary perspective*. Mosby Year Book, Toronto.

Christie-Seeley, I. (1984) *Working with the Family in Primary Care. A Systems Approach to Health and Illness*, p. 4. Praeger, New York.

Clark, P. (1987) Individual autonomy, cooperative empowerment in planning for long term care decision making. *Journal of Aging Studies*, 1(1), 65–76.

Clark, P. (1988) Autonomy, personal empowerment and quality of life in long term care. *The Journal of Applied Gerontology* 7(3), 279–99.

Coulton, C., Dunkle, R., Chow, J., Haug, M., & Vrelhaber, D. (1988) Dimensions of post-hospital care decision making: a factor analytic study. *The Gerontologist*, **28**, 218–23.

Deber, R.B. & Baumann, A.O. (1992) Clinical reasoning in medicine and nursing: decision making versus problem solving. *Teaching and Learning in Medicine*, 4(3), 140–46.

Dubeau, C., Voytovich, A., & Rippey, R. (1986) Premature conclusions in the diagnosis of iron-deficiency anaemia: cause and effect. *Medical Decision Making*, 6(3), 169–73.

Egan, G., & Cowan, M.A. (1979) *People in System: A Model for Development in the Human-Service Professions and Education*. Brooks/Cole, Monterey, CA.

Fozard, J.L. & Costa, P.T. Jr. (1983) Age difference in memory and decision-making in relation to personality, abilities, and endocrine function; Implications for clinical practice and health planning policy. In *Aging: A Challenge to Science and Society*, Vol. 3, (eds J.E. Birren, J.M.A. Munnichs, H. Thomas & M. Marois). Oxford University Press, London.

Gillis, C.L. Highley, B.L., Roberts, B.M. & Martinson, I.M. (1989) *Toward a Science of Family Nursing*. Addison-Wesley, Menlo Park, CA.

Halm, M.A. (1992) Support and reassurance needs: strategies for practice. *Critical Care Nursing Clinics of North America*, 4(4), 633–43.

Hogarth, J. (1978) *Glossary of Health Care Terminology*, p. 143. World Health Organization, Copenhagen.

Holsti, O.R. (1978) Limitations of cognitive abilities in the face of crisis. In *Studies in Crisis Management* (eds C. Smart & W. Standbury), pp. 39–55. Butterworth, Toronto.

Kahneman, D., Slovic, P. & Tverskey, A. (1982) *Judgment Under Uncertainty: Heuristics and Biases*. Cambridge University Press, Cambridge.

Kulys, R. (1983) Future crises and the very old: implications for discharge planning. *Health and Social Work*, **22**, 182–95.

Leavitt, M.B. (1982) *Families at Risk: Primary Prevention in Nursing Practice*. Little, Brown, Boston.

Levkoff, S. & Wetle, T. (1989) Clinical decision making in the care of the aged. *Journal of Aging and Health*, 1(1), 83–101.

March, J. & Simon, H. (1958) *Organizations*. Wiley, New York.

Miller, J.R. (1980–81) Family support of the elderly. *Family and Community Health*, **3**, 39.

Neuman, B. (1974) The Betty Neuman health care systems model: a total approach to patient problems. In *Conceptual Models for Nursing Practice* (eds J.R. Riehl & C. Roy), Appleton-Century–Crofts, Norwalk, Conn.

Neuman, B. (1982) *The Neuman Systems Model: Application to Nursing Education and Practice*. Appleton–Century–Crofts, Norwalk, Connecticut.

Neuman, B. (1989) *The Neuman Systems Model: Application to Nursing Education and Practice*. Appleton–Century–Crofts, Norwalk, Conn.

Phillips, D.C. (1976) *Holistic Thought in Social Science*. Stanford University Press, Palo Alto, CA.

Reed, K. (1989) The Neuman systems model: a basis for family psychosocial assessment and intervention. In *The Neuman Systems Model: Applications to Nursing Education and*

Practice (ed. B. Neuman), pp. 188–95. Appleton–Century– Crofts, Norwalk, Conn.

Simon, H. (1957) *Administrative Behaviour*, 2nd edn. MacMillan, New York.

Thompson, E.H. Jr., Futterman, A.M., Gallagher-Thompson, D., Rose, J.M. & Lovett, S.B. (1993) Social support and caregiving burden in family caregivers of frail elders. *Journal of Gerontology*, 48(5), 245–54.

Wiley, S.D. (1983) Structural treatment application for families in crises: a challenge to rehabilitation. *American Journal of Physical Medicine*, **62**(6), 271–86.

Wright, L.M. & Leahey, M. (1984) *Nurses and Families: A Guide to Family Assessment and Intervention*. F.A. Davis, Philadelphia.

Chapter 12
An evaluation of the Johnson Behavioural System Model of Nursing

WILLIAM REYNOLDS, *RMN, RNT, RGN, MPhil*
Senior Tutor, Highland College of Nursing and Midwifery, Inverness

and DESMOND F.S. CORMACK, *RMN, RGN, MPhil, DipEd, DipN, PhD*
Honorary Reader in Health and Nursing, Queen Margaret College, Edinburgh,
Scotland

In this chapter the authors evaluate the Johnson Behavioural System Model of Nursing by applying the assessment criteria described in an earlier paper. Data for the evaluation were collected by one of the authors (W.R.) at the UCLA Neuropsychiatric Institute and Hospital, and the UCLA School of Nursing, Los Angeles. The major focus of this chapter relates to how nurses at the above facilities apply the Johnson Behavioural System Model of Nursing and how that relates to the questions posed in a previous paper which should be asked by clinicians when assessing the relevance of a model to clinical nursing practice: (a) To what extent does the model assist with the identification of the range of human responses to actual or potential health problems? (b) How does the model enable a nursing diagnosis to be made, and what is the basis of that diagnosis? (c) Does the model explain why individuals respond to health problems in the way that they do? (d) Does the model inform clinicians of the nursing interventions required to enable the client to move towards optimum health? (e) Does the model help to provide an understanding of the desired outcome of nursing intervention? Additionally, new criteria subsequently developed by the authors (Cormack & Reynolds, 1992), and which were not applied here, are proposed for future use in relation to the evaluation of the clinical and practical utility of models used by nurses.

Professional practice

The professional practice of nursing at the University of California, Los Angeles (UCLA) Neuropsychiatric Institute and Hospital is defined as the diagnosis and treatment of human responses to actual or potential health problems (American Nurses' Association, 1980). There, the independent practice of nursing is based on the Johnson Behavioural System Model of Nursing. This theoretical framework is utilized throughout all wards in the hospital, forming the basis for all major nursing decisions in respect to nursing diagnosis, care plans, discharge planning and quality assurance. The Johnson model forms the basis of a primary nursing system which has operated for approximately 12 years. The quality of professional nursing practice is widely recognized as excellent, and characterized by humanistic care based on accountability, autonomy and authority.

A debate which the profession is currently undertaking concerns the applicability and usefulness of nursing models, and the extent to which nursing theory can be said to exist. Some authors such as Luker (1988) have suggested that nursing models may be pretentious theory.

Similar views have been expressed by Loughlin (1988) and Smoyak (1988). Smoyak has also argued that there is no such thing as nursing theory because there is no copyright or ownership of theory. She suggests that nursing, like medicine, is an applied science that borrows knowledge and insight generated by all disciplines, including nursing. While it is possible that nursing models are no more than 'word salads' or metaparadigms consisting of self-evident statements that have little direct relevance to nursing practice, the authors take the view that it is too early to make such a judgement, and that the 'ownership' of theory is a semantic debate. What is important for the nursing profession to know is whether theory-based practice, irrespective of whether it comes from insights generated by nursing or from other disciplines, results in better care or improved health outcomes for clients or patients.

This chapter analyses the Johnson model by applying Reynolds & Cormack's (1990) criteria for assessing the usefulness of nursing theory.

Relevance of a model

Reynolds & Cormack (1990) propose that clinicians should ask the following questions when assessing the relevance of a model to clinical nursing practice:

(1) To what extent does the model assist with the identification of the range of human responses to actual or potential health problems?
(2) How does the model enable a nursing diagnosis to be made, and what is the basis of that diagnosis?
(3) Does the model explain why individuals respond to health problems in the way that they do?
(4) Does the model inform clinicians of the nursing interventions required to enable the client to move towards optimum health?
(5) Does the model help to provide an understanding of the desired outcome of nursing intervention?

These questions were applied to data collected by W.R. in seven wards at the UCLA Neuropsychiatric Institute and Hospital where nursing care is based on the application of the Johnson Behavioural System Model of Nursing.

The Johnson Behavioural System Model of Nursing

The Johnson Behavioural System Model of Nursing is less well known than other models, particularly those of Orem (1985), Roy (1981), Neuman (1989) and Peplau (1988). It has its antecedents in systems theory and has a wide application in that it identifies common patterns of behaviour applicable to all persons regardless of factors such as age and clinical setting. It was selected as the basis for nursing practice at the UCLA Neuropsychiatric Institute and Hospital for three primary reasons. First, it focuses on *observable* behaviours of the patient with which nursing is concerned. Second, it emphasizes the bio-psycho-sociocultural factors which influence behaviour, thereby permitting application in all clinical settings. Third, the model identifies universal patterns of behaviour applicable to all individuals regardless of age, cultural differences or medical diagnosis.

The Johnson model includes the following elements:

(1) The individual is conceptualized as a living system in constant interaction with the environment.
(2) Specific system tasks are carried out by the individual's eight behavioural subsystems. These are the ingestive, eliminative, affiliative, dependency, sexual, aggressive – protective, achievement and restorative subsystems. Although each subsystem has a specific task, the individual is viewed as a whole by virtue of the interdependence of each subsystem (Table 12.1).
(3) Balance is maintained when there is an equal distribution of energy among the eight subsystems. Energy refers to the subsystem's ability to carry out its task adequately.
(4) Environment is viewed as all regulatory elements that influence the behavioural systems such as bio-physical, psychological and developmental status, and sociocultural, family and physical environmental factors. Examples include internal regulators such as cardiovascular functioning or external regulators such as family dynamics.
(5) Observed patient behaviours associated with each of the subsystems are the end product of a complex interaction between bio-psycho-socio regulators specific to that individual, as well as the influence of the immediate situational and environmental factors.
(6) The goal of nursing is to create an environment that nurtures, protects and stimulates the behavioural subsystems so that the individual's system balance is maintained or restored. This could involve helping individuals

Table 12.1 Subsystem definitions (adapted from Dee & Randell (1989) with the authors' permission).

Ingestive
Behaviours associated with the intake of needed resources from the external environment, including food, fluid, information, objects, for the purpose of establishing an effective relationship with the environment.

Eliminative
Behaviours associated with the release of physical waste products.

Affiliative
Behaviours associated with the development and maintenance of interpersonal relationships with parents, peers, authority figures. Establishes a sense of relatedness and belonging with others including attachment behaviours, interpersonal relationships and communication skills.

Dependency
Behaviours associated with obtaining assistance from others in the environment for completing tasks and/or emotional supports. Includes seeking of attention, approval, recognition, basic self-care skills and emotional security.

Sexual
Behaviours associated with a specific gender identify for the purpose of ensuring pleasure/ procreation, and knowledge and behaviour being congruent with biological sex.

Aggressive-protective
Behaviours associated with real or potential threat in the environment for the purpose of ensuring survival. Protection of self through direct or indirect acts. Identification of potential danger.

Achievement
Behaviours associated with mastery of oneself and one's environment for the purpose of producing a desired effect. Includes problem-solving activities. Knowledge of personal strengths and weaknesses.

Restorative
Behaviours associated with maintaining or restoring energy equilibrium, e.g. relief from fatigue, recovery from illness, sleep behaviour, leisure/recreational interests and sick role behaviour.

---

to rest, sleep or develop friendship relationships, depending on the subsystem or the nature of the malfunctions.

To what extent does the model assist with the identification of the range of human responses to actual or potential health problems?

Human responses to actual or potential health problems constitute part of the American Nurses' Association's (ANA's) (1980) definition of the practice of nursing which states that:

'Nursing is the diagnosis and treatment of human responses to potential and actual health problems.'

That definition is also enshrined in the California Nurses' Association's (1989) framework for nursing practice. The four defining characteristics of nursing within the ANA's definition are phenomena, theory, actions and effects. Human responses constitute the *phenomena* which are of concern to, and responsive to, nursing intervention. Examples include alterations in levels of consciousness, self-care limitations, pain and discomfort, physiological defects such as cardiac, respiratory and neurological defects, anxiety, confusion, mood disorders and hallucinations. Phenomena, contained within a diagnostic framework, provide the focus for nursing interventions; nursing diagnosis refers to the practice of identifying and naming the phenomena.

Nurses at the Neuropsychiatric Institute and Hospital did use the diagnostic framework described by the Johnson model to seek and discover the needs of clients that were potentially responsive to nursing actions. Although this approach could be criticized on the grounds that nurses were attempting to fit clinical data into contrived categories, the problems identified were arguably good examples of clients' attempts to maintain their health in a manner which was often ineffectual, or which further damaged their health status. Examples included denial of illness, overeating, auditory hallucinations, hostility and negative self-concept.

How does the model enable a nursing diagnosis to be made, and what is the basis of that diagnosis?

Nursing diagnosis refers to the naming of patients' health problems which are of concern to nurses, and which are responsive to nursing intervention. It refers to the phenomena to which the skills of nurses must be applied in order to bring about favourable health outcomes for their patients. One of the purported advantages of the Johnson model is that it makes a contribution to the development of a nursing diagnostic system. Dee & Randell (1989) suggest that it delineates nursing's distinct contribution to care.

Making a nursing diagnosis using the Johnson model involves several distinct phases, each requiring an increasingly greater level of nursing knowledge, experience and clinical skills. The route consists of the following steps. The first involves the identification of malfunction in any of the subsystems, and placing observed behaviours into the correct subsystem; for example, sleeping during the daytime and/or periodic awakening during the night indicates a problem with the restorative subsystem. At this point it is simply a restorative subsystem problem. The second step is to determine from the behavioural data the effectiveness of each subsystem; that is, to ask how effective the subsystem is in achieving its purpose (see Table 12.1).

The third step involves the search for environmental regulators that are impacting upon any of the client's subsystems. At this stage, nursing diagnoses are based on the demonstration of ineffective behaviour within one or more subsystems, and the relationship of these behaviours to the regulators. For example, an adolescent who has verbal conflict with his peers, steals, teases or interrupts others' conversation, has a problem with the dependency subsystem where, according to Johnson (1980), the goal is to seek approval, attention and recognition. Further study of the client's environment reveals that the parents are divorced, that he lives with his mother who is clinically depressed and states that she cannot manage the son's behaviour. This suggests that the family circumstances are regulating, impacting on, the dependency subsystem. Essentially, the search for the regulators of subsystem behaviour is the equivalent to the search for the aetiology of behaviour.

Finally, a complete nursing diagnosis is made. This involves making a statement which describes the nature of the subsystem problem, particularly in respect to the relationship of one subsystem behaviour to another. Currently, nurses at this hospital are working with several diagnostic labels which describe the nature of the subsystem problem; these are insufficiency, discrepancy, dominance and incompatibility of the subsystem (see Table 12.2).

If a subsystem is disturbed it will always be possible to make a simple subsystem diagnosis such as insufficiency or discrepancy of the ingestive subsystem. Less experienced nurses are likely to generate frequent single subsystem diagnoses. However, nurses need to ask themselves if the behaviour in one subsystem is related in any way to inefficient behaviour in another subsystem; for example, dominance of the aggressive–protective

Table 12.2 Criteria for diagnostic labels (adapted from Dee & Randell (1989) with the authors' permission).

	Criteria
Insufficiency	A diagnosis of insuffiency implies that the subsystem is underdeveloped, lacking in capacity and unable to function normally.
Discrepancy	A diagnosis of discrepancy means the behaviour within a subsystem is different from or at variance with the goal of that sybsystem.
Dominance	A diagnosis of dominance means the behaviour within one subsystem is overdeveloped, and prevails over other subsystems, outweighing in influence and effect.
Incompatibility	A diagnosis of incompatibility means that the subsystem behaviours exhibited to meet the goal of one subsystem are incongruent/antagonistic with the behaviour exhibited to meet the goal of another subsystem.

subsystem over the affiliative subsystem – that is, a two-system diagnosis. If the answer is yes, there is a need to determine whether the observed behaviour is better explained, understood and responded to if it is described in a diagnosis which pairs it with another subsystem.

Making a nursing diagnosis

As with all hospitals, the Neuropsychiatric Institute and Hospital has a staff group with varying levels of experiences, qualifications, ability and diagnostic skills. At the time this visit was undertaken, 33% of nursing staff held a master's degree, 5% were doctorally prepared, and 50% held a BSN (Bachelor of Science in Nursing) degree. The following anecdote constitutes, in the view of the writers, a skilled application of the diagnostic aspect of the Johnson Behavioural System Model to making a *nursing* diagnosis of a young Mexican boy who had been *medically* diagnosed as suffering from terminal cancer.

The behavioural characteristics of the clinical data with which this child presented included refusal to eat and marked weight loss, accompanied with minimal verbalization. Previously, he had had a history of fighting frequently with other children and had made threats of self-harm that had not materialized thus far. A staff nurse emphasized the degree of clinical thinking necessary to make an accurate Johnson diagnosis, and the basis for making that diagnosis. She reported:

> 'It would be easy to view the problem as being insufficiency of the ingestive subsystem, but to arrive at an accurate diagnosis you really need to know the goal of the patient. This involves an examination of the relationship between subsystem malfunction and bio-psycho-socio regulators.
>
> Often the patient's goals regarding behaviour are associated with cultural norms. For example, the Mexican boy came with expectations and cultural norms acquired from his Hispanic culture. Eating is considered to be a major event in that culture; it is a source of enjoyment and a family group activity. My view was that non-compliance with eating was his way of taking control over an area of his life. This was important because he was facing the prospect of increased helplessness and dependency on others. Taking control and being in charge *was the goal for this patient*. The nursing diagnosis was incompatibility of the achievement subsystem and the aggressive–protective subsystem.
>
> Looking at his previous behaviour, fighting with peers, there is a need to ask why he was getting into fights. The *why* is the *regulator*, that is what fighting is related to. The answer could be that it is a socio-cultural norm, a learned behaviour. The weight loss contributed to his inability to do things for himself in the ways that were learned from his culture.

Inexperienced staff tend to take a concrete and step-by-step approach to diagnosis. Staff who pay attention to the client's affective state seem to be more effective in knowing where to put behaviours, and what these behaviours mean.'

It could be suggested that this degree of insight into the purpose of the client's coping behaviours occurred in spite of the model; that is, as a consequence of high empathy nursing. However, while cause–effect relationships are difficult to establish, the following case conference does support the argument that the model encouraged nurses to make a nursing diagnosis, and link that diagnosis to environmental regulators of behaviour.

Case conference (summary)

This conference occurred in an adolescent unit. It concerned a young woman who lived apart from her parents but whose recent behaviour had been causing them some concern. The *medical* diagnosis was florid psychosis. A discussion took place about what would constitute a suitable *nursing* diagnosis. The nursing opinion was that, in response to environmental stressors, the patient characteristically responded impulsively.

Environmental stressors were identified as loneliness, lack of achievement at work, and failure in relationships with significant others including parents. Impulsive behaviours were defined as excessive alcohol consumption, drug taking and choosing inappropriate relationships. The view was that the capacity to live independently was threatened by her inability to protect herself. Thus, the human responses to potential health problems were further threatening her health status. The full nursing diagnosis which eventually emerged was incompatibility of the aggressive–protective and achievement subsystems.

The authors concluded that the Johnson model does enable a nursing diagnosis to be made, and enable nurses to describe the basis of that diagnosis.

Does the model explain why individuals respond to health problems in the way that they do?

In parallel with making a nursing diagnosis, the 'what' of problem identification, there is a need to explain the individual's response to health problems, the 'why' of diagnosis. Implicit in the Johnson diagnostic system is the need to determine whether there is a single or multiple system malfunction. If more than one is involved, the nurse establishes whether the problem results from one dominating the other(s) or from the goal of one being antagonistic to that of another. If only one subsystem is involved, the nurse establishes if the problem is one of insufficiency (under-development of the system function) or discrepancy (subsystem behaviour at variance with its goals).

Next, the reason for the subsystem(s) malfunction is identified in terms of the influencing environmental factors being identified. These factors, referred to as regulators, include family dynamics, past learning or physical disabilities. They represent the aetiology of the problem in the same way as famine (the regulator) causes malnutrition (the problem). Such regulators can be external (for example, family issues, such as finance or alcohol abuse) or internal (anxiety, for example). Thus, the Johnson model provides nurses with the means with which to explain why individuals respond to health problems in the way that they do.

Does the model inform clinicians of the nursing interventions required to enable the client to move towards optimum health?

Having made an accurate diagnosis and explained the individual's responses to health problems, the nurse then needs to decide which nursing interventions will enable the client to move towards optimum health. What is of interest to all nurses is the extent to which a particular model provides clues, or enables them to select and implement nursing interventions which are appropriate to the particular circumstances of the patient. Unless nursing interventions have a theoretical underpinning they may, at best, be inappropriate. At worse, they can harm the patient. It was concluded that whilst the Johnson model was an effective diagnostic tool, in the sense of answering the question 'Why do people do the things that they do?', it did not specify or prescribe consequent nursing actions. The Johnson model is an incomplete theoretical statement because it does not specify links between diagnosis and intervention. In short, it does not provide a direct link between diagnosis and intervention.

Whilst it is arguable that the Johnson model provides clues for intervention – for example, it may focus the nurse's attention on family issues and the possible need for family therapy – it does not delineate the specific interventions required to promote optimum health for the patient. Although nurses at the UCLA Neuropsychiatric Institute and Hospital valued the diagnostic focus offered by the model, it was observed that subsequent interventions emanated from other models and theories such as client-centred therapy, cognitive therapy, behavioural therapy, general systems theory and Peplau's interpersonal theory. Theories borrowed from other disciplines were then reshaped into a manner applicable to nursing. A head nurse who agreed with this conclusion expressed it thus:

'The goal of nursing is to search for and understand the regulators of the client's behaviour; then we select interventions from the literature.'

Nursing care plans

An interesting feature of the nursing approach at this hospital is the existence of standardized nursing care plans. At the time of the visit, approximately 30 were in use, and more were being developed. These care plans, which were individualized when applied to specific patients, had their origins in the literature and inductive theory resulting from clinical practice at this hospital. Phenomena addressed by existing standardized care plans included stereotypic behaviours, self-injurious behaviour, bizarre speech, clinging/over-attention to adults, stealing, smearing faeces, inappropriate intentional urinating, poor self-esteem, inability to make friends, and so on. Many of the interventions appeared to stem from behavioural therapy methodology, and included limit setting, time out, ignoring and positive/negative reinforcement for maladaptive behaviours.

Thus, nurses were using the Johnson model to make a nursing diagnosis, and other theoretical statements to identify appropriate interventions. This supported Smoyak's (1988) view that nursing is an applied rather than a pure science. Examination of the clinical application of the Johnson model indicates that it does not enable nurses to define or prescribe appropriate nursing interventions relating to a specific nursing diagnosis.

Does the model help to provide an understanding of the desired outcome of nursing intervention?

This final question relates to the extent to which a model enables nurses to make statements about hypothesized links between nursing input and health outcomes for patients. This involves an understanding of the desired outcome of nursing interventions.

Auger & Dee (1982, 1983) present evidence supporting the efficacy of the Johnson model as a tool for evaluating nursing interventions. These authors developed the UCLA Neuropsychiatric Institute and Hospital Patient Classification System which is based on the Johnson Behavioural System Model of Nursing. In contrast to previously existing patient classification systems designed specifically for administrative purposes, Auger & Dee's system is integrated with the nursing process and is expressly intended to be used as a clinical measure of patient progress, in addition to the administrative determination of staffing levels.

The work of Auger & Dee led to the development of behavioural indices, with each subsystem operationalized in terms of critical adaptive and maladaptive behaviours. The behaviours were ranked into categories according to their assumed level of adaptiveness. A panel of expert clinicians rated each behaviour for compliance with an acuity rating scale of 1 to 4. Nursing intervention derived from an analysis of existing care plans were also ranked according to the frequency, intensity and nature of nursing contact. As with client behaviours, these were rated between 1 and 4 (Table 12.3).

Based on the behavioural data, each subsystem is assigned a behavioural category score ranging from 1 to 4 (1 = effective: 2 = inconsistently effective: 3 = ineffective: 4 = severely ineffective). These scores are in effect an acuity rating and provide some basis for allocating nursing resources. That is possible because the severity of the illness is manifested behaviourally and this reflects the degree of difficulty in nursing the patient and the consequent type of clinical skills needed. For example, category 4 refers to behaviours that are incompatible with the subsystem's goal.

Taking the aggressive–protective subsystem as an example, where the goal is self-protection and preservation, a level of 4 might indicate a very high suicidal or self-harm potential. Therefore, a client assessed as having a level 4 acuity rating would require continuous one-to-one nursing and a suicide prevention plan. The resource implications are that the patient requires a continuous presence of a nurse who has the experience and clinical ability necessary for the prevention of self-harm, and the client is assessed as being at level 4. That level of nursing care is required until the client's acuity level changes, for example to level 1. The criteria for rating client's behaviour categories, and the levels of nursing intervention required for each category, are outlined in Table 12.3

Despite the difficulties experienced in establishing cause–effect relationships in multidisciplinary care settings, this tool does provide the basis for answering the question 'Does nursing make any difference?' It also provides a basis for planning the skills mix required by the nursing service, and the quality assurance programmes

Conclusion

During the initial evaluation of the clinical applicability of the Johnson Behavioural System Model of Nursing, the model was evaluated against five criteria developed by Reynolds & Cormack (1990). Whilst the model met some of these criteria, it did not provide clear answers to others. The relatively weak aspect of this model is its inability to identify or prescribe specific nursing interventions. It was also suggested that the links between levels of acuity, nursing input and outcome, established by UCLA Neuropsychiatric Institute and Hospital, require comment and validation by the international nursing community. It is possible that if the extended

Table 12.3   UCLA Neuropsychiatric Hospital Nursing Department criteria for rating patient behaviour categories and levels of nursing interventions (adapted from Dee & Randell (1989) with the authors' permission).

Categories of patient behaviour	Levels of nursing intervention
Category 1 Patient demonstrates behaviours/actions that are effective and compatible in all eight subsystems, therefore achieving system balance. Energy may be unequally distributed among the eight subsystems but not to the detriment of any one subsystem or to the system as a whole. System balance denotes health.	*Level 1* Category 1 patients demonstrate system balance; therefore they are able to protect, nurture and stimulate all behavioural subsystems. The patient requires a minimum amount of nursing time in supervision and nursing care. The primary goal of nursing care for the category 1 patient is the provision of a nurturing and stimulating environment within a group context.
Category 2 Patient demonstrates behaviours/actions that are inconsistently effective in one or more subsystem(s), resulting in short-term incompatibility among the subsystems and the potential for system imbalance. Energy may be temporarily distributed unequally among the subsystems creating ineffective subsystem functioning but not to the detriment of the system as a whole. Potential for system imbalance results in the potential for health deviation.	*Level 2* Category 2 patients demonstrate a potential for system imbalance; therefore they are not able to consistently protect, nurture and stimulate all behavioural subsystems. The patient requires a moderate amount of nursing time in supervision and nursing care. The primary goal of nursing care for the category 2 patient is the provision of a nurturing, stimulating and protective environment within a group context.
Category 3 Patient demonstrates behaviours/actions that are incompatible with one or more subsystems resulting in system imbalance and incompatibility among subsystems. Energy is unequally distributed among the eight subsystems and frequently results in the detriment of the system as a whole. System imbalance results in illness.	*Level 3* Category 3 patients demonstrate system imbalance; therefore they are not able to protect, nurture and stimulate all behavioural subsystems. The patient requires an intensive amount of nursing time in supervision and care. The primary goal of nursing care for the category 3 patient is the provision of a nurturing and protective environment on an individual level or within a small group.
Category 4 Patient demonstrates behaviours/actions that are highly incompatible with one or more subsystems, resulting in system imbalance and severe incompatibility among the subsystems that threatens survival. Energy is unequally distributed among the subsystems and this distribution of energy is of such acute intensity, long duration and/or high frequency that detriment to the system as a whole is evident. Severe system imbalance results in critical illness.	*Level 4* Category 4 patients demonstrate severe system imbalance; therefore they are not able to protect, nurture and stimulate all behavioural subsystems. The patient requires continuous one-to-one supervision and nursing care. The primary goal of nursing care for the category 4 patient is the provision of a nurturing and protective environment on an individual level.

criteria proposed in this chapter were to be applied to the Johnson model, further limitations to its clinical usefulness and applicability would be detected.

A major issue facing the nursing profession relating to the clinical applicability of nursing theories concerns the extent to which deductive theories, such as the Johnson model, are preferable to inductively developed theories of nursing which include the development of a diagnostic taxonomy produced from the expressed concerns of clients, and which nurses observe during nurse–client interactions. Thus, such a diagnostic taxonomy would develop from expressed and observed needs rather than cause the nurse to fit clinical data into global theoretical frameworks which may have a limited actual clinical basis. Peplau (1986), cited by Reynolds & Cormack (1990), suggests that clinical data derived from observations of human responses to health threats have explanatory powers and provide the basis for the development and testing of nursing theory.

Further evaluation

Subsequent to this evaluation of the Johnson behavioural model it became clear that the evaluation criteria (questions) used required further development, and that further criteria could have been profitably applied. These further criteria for evaluating the clinical and practical utility of models were presented in papers by Cormack & Reynolds (1992) and Reynolds (1993). These works resulted from the authors' experience in evaluating the Johnson model and from experiences with clinical nurses who were striving to answer the question 'Does this or that theory or model have any practical utility in my clinical practice?' In particular, we shared the view that all models used by nurses needed to be subjected to a much wider and more rigorous range of evaluation criteria than had previously been the case. It is proposed, therefore, that the following additional questions should be posed in relation to all models when evaluating their clinical and practical utility.

First, is the extent of the scope (focus) of the model clearly delineated in terms of the client group to which it applies? Because nurses deliver care to a very diverse group of clients it is questionable if models with, for example, a unitary focus such as systems theory, self care deficiency, interpersonal relations, can be applied to the needs and copying strategies of *all* client groups. In spite of claims made by Johnson theorists that the model has a wide theoretical application, our view is that doubts persist about the universal applicability of the model to *all* client groups.

Further questions developed by the authors, but not applied to the Johnson model, relate to the extent to which models are reliable and valid. Reliability refers to the extent to which clinicians are enabled to reach agreement in the way that they perceive clients with identical nursing needs. Validity refers to the extent to which skilled nurse users of a model are able to identify similar nursing diagnoses and intervention in clients with identical nursing needs.

Language can be a barrier

Further important issues are the extent to which the model is culturally and geographically portable, and the extent to which the description, structure, content and application of the model can be understood by nurse clinicians. Whilst physicians can usually understand each other's professional language nationally and internationally, we propose that this is not so in nursing. This was brought to the attention of one of the authors (W.R.) when a UCLA nurse informed him that nurses in another Los Angeles hospital (where she worked part-time) would not be able to understand the language of the Johnson model. It seems that language can act as a barrier to communication among nurses in the same town/city, as well as internationally.

Clinicians are, rightly, increasingly concerned about the ethical aspects of models application, and feel it reasonable to expect model creators to ensure that models are 'ethical' and to fully address this issue when describing the model. Furthermore, clinicians expect models to provide them with an approach to nursing which is consistent with the notion of clinical autonomy.

An additional and important aspect of model evaluation, and one which clinicians also expect model creators to address, is the extent to which the theoretical constructs which constitute the model have been tested and accepted. For example some UCLA nurses emphasized the centrality of the aggressive/protective subsystem within the Johnson model. By this they meant that changes within this subsystem cause changes in other subsystems. This hypothesized cause–effect relationship in our view requires further exploration (see also Derdiarian, 1990).

Educative clinical experience

Whilst the process of validating models would be facilitated if creators of nursing models addressed issues regarding practical and clinical utility, this process is also dependent on clinicians' critical reasoning. This involves the ability to see things afresh and to be sensitive to the limits of existing information, an ability which is somewhat analagous to cognitive–behavioural empathy. Some writers suggest that this skill is best learned during educative *clinical experience* followed by supervised review of inter-action data with a skilled teacher (Peplau, 1986; Reynolds, 1990). This proposition is currently being studied (by W.R.) in relation to registered nurses' empathy.

Acknowledgement

The authors wish to acknowledge the friendliness and help experienced by W. Reynolds from the nursing staff of the UCLA Neuropsychiatric Hospital and the Nursing Faculty of the UCLA School of Nursing, during a visit to Los Angeles in May 1990.

References

American Nurses' Association (1980) *Nursing: A Social Policy Statement*. American Nurses' Association, Kansas. City.

Auger, J. & Dee, V. (1982) Can a nursing model be translated into clinical practice? *Paper presented at National Symposium of Nursing Research, San Francisco, 19 November*.

Auger, J. & Dee, V. (1983) A patient classification system based on the Behavioral System Model of Nursing: Part 1. *The Journal of Nursing Administration*, **13**(4), 38–43.

California Nurses' Association (1989) *Nursing Practice in California, Rights, Responsibilities and Regulations*, 2nd edn. California Nurses' Association, San Francisco.

Cormack, D. & Reynolds , W. (1992) Criteria for evaluating the clinical and practical utility of models used by nurses. *Journal of Advanced Nursing*, **17**, 1472–8.

Dee, V. & Randell, B. (1989) *N.P.H. Patient Classification System: Theory-Based Nursing Practice Model for Staffing*. Nursing Department, UCLA Neuropsychiatric Institute and Hospital, Los Angeles.

Derdiarian, A. (1990) The relationships among the subsystems of Johnson's Behavioural System model. *Image: Journal of Nursing Scholarship*, **22**, 219–25.

Johnson, D.E. (1980) The Behavioural System Model for Nursing. In *Conceptual Models for Nursing Practice* (eds J.P. Riehl & C. Roy) 2nd edn. Appleton–Century–Crofts, New York.

Loughlin, K. (1988) Modelled, muddled and befuddled. *Nursing Times*, **84**(5), 30–31.

Luker, K. (1988) Do models work? *Nursing Times*, **88**(5), 27–9.

Neuman, B. (1989) *The Neuman Systems Model*, 2nd edn. Appleton & Lange, Norwalk, Connecticut.

Orem, D. (1985) *Nursing: Concepts of Practice*, 3rd edn. McGraw-Hill, New York.

Peplau, H. (1986) *Psychiatric Nursing Skills: Today and Tomorrow – A World Overview*. Paper presented at a Celebration of Skills, Third International Congress of Psychiatric Nursing, Imperial College, London, September.

Peplau, H. (1988) *Interpersonal Relations in Nursing*. Macmillan, London.

Reynolds, W. (1990) Teaching psychiatric and mental health nursing: a teaching perspective. In *Psychiatric and Mental Health Nursing: Theory and Practice* (eds. W. Reynolds & D. Cormack). Chapman and Hall, London.

Reynolds, W. (1993) Criteria to evaluate nursing theories and models. *Journal of Psychosocial Nursing*, Nov. (editorial).

Reynolds, W. & Cormack, D. (eds) (1990) Psychiatric and mental health nursing: theory and practice. In *Psychiatric and Mental Health Nursing: Theory and Practice* (eds. W. Reynolds & D. Cormack), pp. 3–22. Chapman & Hall, London.

Roy, C. (1981) *Theory Construction in Nursing: An Adaptation Model*. Appleton & Lange, Norwalk, Connecticut.

Smoyak, S. (1988) Strategies for theory development. *Proceedings: Fifth Nursing Science Colloquim*. Boston University School of Nursing, Boston.

Acknowledgements

The chapters in this book are updated papers originally published in the *Journal of Advanced Nursing*. Listed below are references to the original versions.

1 *Problems with paradigms in a caring profession* by Jane J.A. Robinson: *Journal of Advanced Nursing* (1992) **17**, 632–8. This was based on a paper delivered as part of a seminar series on Art and Science in Nursing held at the Institute of Nursing, Radcliffe Infirmary, Oxford, 28 February 1991.

2 *Concepts, analysis and the development of nursing knowledge: the evolutionary cycle* by Beth L. Rodgers: *Journal of Advanced Nursing* (1989) **14**, 330–35.

3 *Restructuring: an emerging theory on the process of losing weight* by Rosemary Johnson: *Journal of Advanced Nursing* (1990) **15**, 1289–96.

4 *Benevolence, a central moral concept derived from a grounded theory study of nursing decision making in psychiatric settings* by Kim Lützén and Conny Nordin: *Journal of Advanced Nursing* (1993) **18**, 1106–11.

5 *Mid-range theory building and the nursing theory–practice gap: a respite care case study* by Mike Nolan and Gordon Grant: *Journal of Advanced Nursing* (1992) **17**, 217–23.

6 *Toward a theory of touch: the touching process and acquiring a touching style* by Carole A. Estabrooks and Janice M. Morse: *Journal of Advanced Nursing* (1992) **17**, 448–56.

7 *Can combined oral contraceptives be made more effective by means of a nursing care model?* by Marianne Lindell and Henny Olsson: *Journal of Advanced Nursing* (1991) **16**, 475–9.

8 *Advice concerning breastfeeding from mothers of infants admitted to a neonatal intensive care unit: the Roy Adaptation Model as a conceptual structure* by Kerstin Hedberg Nyqvist and Per-Olow Sjödén: *Journal of Advanced Nursing* (1993) **18**, 54–63.

9 *Mitral valve prolapse and its effects: a programme of inquiry within Orem's Self-Care Deficit Theory of Nursing* by Sharon William Utz and Mary Carol Ramos: *Journal of Advanced Nursing* (1993) **18**, 742–51. An earlier version of this chapter was presented at the Fourth Annual Conference of the Southern Nursing Research Society, 1990, Orlando, Florida.

10 *The Betty Neuman Systems Model applied to practice: a client with multiple sclerosis* by Janet B. Knight: *Journal of Advanced Nursing* (1990) **15**, 447–55.

11 *The ageing family in crisis: assessment and decision-making models* by Ann C. Beckingham and Andrea Baumann: *Journal of Advanced Nursing* (1990) **15**, 782–7.

12 *An evaluation of the Johnson Behavioural System Model of Nursing* by William Reynolds and Desmond F.S. Cormack: *Journal of Advanced Nursing* (1991) **16**, 1122–30.

Index